Keep your Sacrum more Sacred

An holistic journey through the body to the sacrum

by Gabriele Gad

Second Edition 2010
First published in 2001 by the Author.
An earlier edition was first published under the title *Energy in Balance*

ISBN: 978-1-4457-2637-3

Copyright © Gabriele Gad, 2010

Typesetting and cover design by
David Spofforth

Special thanks go to my dear friend, Jacqueline Lightband for a great deal of help in editing this book and to my husband, David.

Contents

Introduction   iii
What is Balance?   v

The Legs   1
Ground Your Feet   1
Release the Blocked Energy in Your Legs   8

Arms and Heart   12
Balance the Energies in Your Hands   12
The Tina Story   15
Love From the Heart to the Hands   25

The Neck and Shoulders   38
Release the Tension in Shoulders and Neck   38

The Head   45
The Eyes: The Windows of the Soul   45
The Ears: Listening to the Waves   51
The Mouth   54

Keeping Your Sacrum More Sacred   75
Sacrum, Pelvis and Lower Back   75
About Breathing   81
Sexual Issues   88

Energy in Balance   96
Massage of the Head   98

References   78

Introduction

While finishing my diploma in Psychology in Munich I became quite frustrated about the headiness of the subject. Many of the students were intellectuals and we were mostly learning how to test people, how to give them strange names for symptoms that nearly everybody seemed to have experienced anyway.

Thus I started to have Bioenergetic Therapy. Bioenergetic exercises and deep massage on the pelvis then helped me to feel my body much more.

I played the piano in a jazz band and I really wanted to sing as well. The right to sing was mostly kept by the men in the front line who were playing the trumpet, the trombone and the clarinet (The clarinetist was then my husband). They were allowed to present themselves on the stage but I was told that my voice was too high and too thin.

Secretly with my household money I went to see an expensive singing teacher. He showed me how to deepen and increase the volume of my voice by breathing into the lower back. Thus I started singing in public. I learnt that singing exercises and deep massage on bones and muscles were an immense help to find out more about my body and my sexuality.

As a member of the National Federation of Spiritual Healers (NFSH), I have been taught a lot about healing by polish clairvoyant Lilla Bek. Later in life Paula Garbuck's system of 'ring muscle exercises' and the sessions with my therapist Ayelet Amitai were another great help in finding out more about the sacrum and its connection with the body.

As I am sitting here in Vauxhall at my new computer, trying to reshape the book which once was called *Energy in Balance*, I am already excited about my workshop on the sacrum that I am going to give next week at the Mind body spirit festival in the Horticultural Halls. I feel very privileged that I was asked to do this workshop again after it had been sold out last time.

It has always puzzled me, that the backbone on the bottom of our spine has been called the 'sacrum'. Is it really a sacred bone? Does the name stem from ancient times of sacrifice where you were supposed to make love to the temple priest to ask the gods to give you a good harvest for the next year?

As a psychologist who has studied Biodynamic Psychotherapy[1], a body mind therapy based on the teachings of Psychoanalyst Wilhelm Reich and Psychologist Gerda Boyesen, I have always been interested in the function of the pelvis, not just as the centre of support but also as the secret origin of divine energy. I wanted to find out more about the sacredness of the pelvis.

Last but not least Philosopher Rudolf Steiner and his teaching have had a big influence on my life and work.

Trying to bring those different theories together hasn't always been easy. In the last 20 years I have developed a system of workshops starting with feet and hands the so-called exits of the body via the head, the eyes, ears and the mouth. The mouth and the pelvis and genitals are having a lot in common as you will find out later when we look at the system of our 'ring-muscles'.

The workshop on sacrum and sexuality was the workshop people were attending most. But you shouldn't have the cake at the beginning of the meal. It is not good to go to the sacrum straight away. We will approach it gradually following the energy moving through our legs, arms and head towards the trunk via heart, abdomen and sacrum. The first chapter of this book will be on how to look after our feet and how to ground ourselves.

I want to share with you my experience in seven natural ways of healing. Once you know how to use these seven tools on yourself and on others you will start to live your life more consciously and joyfully.

---

[1] In Biodynamic Psychotherapy I learnt how to bring the body and the mind together. The use of the flower and gem essences helped my clients and me immensely to learn to know our different negative states of mind and their connection with the body.

1. Vocal expression and Counseling
2. Creative expression
3. Breathing
4. Exercises (Bioenergetics, Ringmuscle and other exercises)
5. Biodynamic Self and Partner Massage
6. Flower and Gem Essences
7. Spiritual Healing

Please be careful when doing the exercises and take full responsibility for your own safety.

What is Balance?

The first image you might see, if you are thinking about balance could perhaps be a set of old fashioned scales. To achieve a balance, you have to put the same amount of weight on both sides of the scales.

Visualize Leonardo da Vinci's symmetrical man his arms and legs stretched out and think of your own body. Compare the feeling in your right and left hand, your right and left foot. Is there any difference? Do you feel symmetrical like Leonardo's man?

And what about your head and your feet? Is there more energy in your head or in your feet? Do you breathe with an open mouth? And how deep is your breath? If you want to balance yourself, all these things will matter! Are your neck, shoulders or back stiff while you are reading these lines and do you wear glasses?

Some years ago Sabine Kurjo asked me to give a talk on 'Energy in Balance' in the Mandeer, an Indian restaurant where she had arranged weekly talks about alternative therapies. I kept the title for the first edition of my book.

It seems as if the most natural ways to heal our body and mind are hardly practised any more. Things that used to happen naturally such as touch, hands-on -healing, breathing and the use of flowers and stones get more and more forgotten. People want fast cures without having to make any efforts to understand their emotions and their bodies.

Time has become a scarce commodity to most of us, apart from those who are on the dole. And they quite often take drugs (smoking, alcohol, too much food, etc). They tend to use the precious time to look for a job and get into a nervous rush mostly feeling guilty and inadequate. Only a few see the big chance in their life to give some energy and attention to their 'inner child' and to their body after years of abusing it.

'Energy in Balance' means that we are striving towards a balance in our life in many different ways. Balance in various activities acted out with different parts of our body can be an important aim.

Balance in giving and taking is essential. Symmetrical balance within the body especially where we have pairs of limbs and organs is a goal that must have been in Leonardo da Vinci's mind. He was a master of many arts.

Nowadays we usually train to be good in one subject and then we have to perform it for the rest of our lives. Sometimes we are able to have a second subject as a hobby. Usually the pressure to earn money does not leave us with time for anything else. The ambition to be good plays another vital role in people's inhibition to learn things they have always wanted to do.

Leonardo da Vinci's picture of the symmetrical man is a beautiful image for the idea of the energies in the body being in perfect balance. Often the earth is compared with the human body and they both have a lot in common. Meridians in the body correspond to leylines, chakras to places of high energy on the globe, blood vessels and rivers have things in common, the weather can be compared with our emotions just to name a few.

When I was searching for a picture to illustrate the flyers for my workshops I had the idea to use a photograph of a person standing with both arms lifted symmetrically in front of the globe. I have always been fascinated about the idea of finding a balance in my life on different levels. One reason why I joined the Steiner Society was that many members seemed to strive for not just one way to express themselves creatively but several ways. They would learn how to play an instrument, try to write articles and poetry and paint as well. They usually would not try to use their gifts for commercial purposes but save them for their own pleasure balance and for further insights.

I do not think that I want to use just one of my talents and concentrate on bringing it to perfection because that would usually lead me into imbalance. I would start to overuse some parts of my body and neglect the other parts. So, many times in my life people have said to me that I should concentrate on one thing and try to become famous or earn money with it. But it has never really appealed to me to work hard and thus neglect my inner balance. Furthermore I realized that as soon as I was starting to concentrate on earning money the component of having fun could easily disappear. That probably has happened to many people. At first they really enjoyed their work and then gradually it became more and more boring because they always had to do the same things. But they decided to sacrifice the joy to earn money and becoming famous. The Ego crept in and took their fun away and they would usually say "Well, I really have no choice because I have to earn a living and pay the mortgage and I cannot find another job."

I am aware of the fact that I have probably sacrificed my need to earn money and become famous to the need to keep a balance, enjoy my work and have time to learn other important things as well. No money in the world can turn me into a composer, or help me to have time and awareness to understand and study books or learn a new instrument. We should never stop learning new things and visiting classes. It will keep us young and flexible.

To find a balance within our body we can at first look at the pairs of limbs and organs that we have got and find out how to balance them. In the first chapters I start to focus on the feet, the hands, the arms, the eyes and the ears.

viii *Keep your Sacrum more Sacred*

The Legs

When people come to a body-mind workshop they are usually a bit scared. They know that they will not just sit in a circle on chairs and talk. They know that they might be expected to take off some clothes. They might touch someone or be touched by another person. Especially in a workshop where women and men are mixed this can create tension or fear.

As a workshop leader I try to check out at the beginning what the participants are like. Would they dare to take off their socks? Would they lie on a mattress or blanket on the floor? Or would they rather work in a sitting position?

The sacrum lies well hidden at a place that newcomers usually would not want to be touched or exposed. The Biodynamic principle is based on the fact that energy moves in and out the arms and legs. Thus fingers and toes are the doors to the body.

That's why we start our journey with the feet and toes.

Ground Your feet

Why would we want to be grounded? Most of us have too much energy in our heads, because we are thinking too much. Many of us find it difficult to relax and stop thinking. What has happened? The energy might be all blocked inside the head not wanting to go down anymore into the rest of our body. Grounding our feet is one way to get the energy back into the body.

Slavonic sculptor Marco Pogacnik works as a healer of landscapes where the energies have been disturbed. He can really see the nature spirits.

With singing, visualisation and a lot of love he has helped the elemental kingdom in great many ways to recover.

In his book Elemental Beings he refers to 'our elemental I' (I write about it later and call it 'the inner child') who is serving us. He recommends that we should work towards a conscious relationship with this true elemental being.

Marco can see that most of us are taken over by mental patterns and that we have formed a culture concentrated in the head. Thus we are lifted off the ground dwelling on an abstract level of thought.

To get out of this illusionary state and be able to anchor our soulforces in our body as a source of healing and harmony we urgently need 'grounding and earthing'.

He recommends an exercise that can help with the process of grounding:

Focus your awareness on a point below the coccyx to connect yourself with your elemental 'I'. Then concentrate on the middle of your belly and without loosing the connection with the 'earth sphere' bring it up to the belly into the middle of the feeling area from where it can flood through your whole body.

Then concentrate on the area above the head to get in touch with your soul-force (higher or inner self). Now lower this soul experience down into the middle of your heart and let it radiate from there through your whole being.

Imagine that both focal points of your being are harmoniously in tune with each other.

Fashion has always made it difficult for women to be grounded. Wearing high heels with pointed fronts does not allow any energy to move through toes and heels. Stockings made from synthetic materials won't let the legs and feet 'breathe'. Women who usually are wearing short, tight skirts in the cold season might already be used to feeling cold or numb in their feet, legs and buttocks.

It doesn't help that in many English Schools the pupils are usually wearing socks in Winter when they do sport.

Men often have a habit of wearing their boots all the time. Thus the feet never have a chance to breathe. As soon as athlete's feet develop, people feel ashamed of the smell and it makes things even worse.

This brings us to the first tool we are going to use, Biodynamic Self-massage.

Foot Massage

I hope that you will, while you are reading this, be courageous enough to take your shoes and socks off. We are going to massage our own feet. It is important to sit in a comfortable and straight position, where we can breathe deeply. Try to breathe through your mouth all the time. That will help the massage to have a deeper effect on your body.

Toes are the main exits for our energies. Through them energy is travelling out and in just as through doors. The feet are doing a lot of work for us all through the day. But very seldom we are thinking of giving them any attention. Let's think of our toes as children who might want some of our attention before they will claim it through tension and pain. You can use some oil or cream, if you wish, almond oil mixed with lavender oil for example.

When you massage your toe it is good to imagine, that the energy that you are using for thinking is travelling down from your head, down the arms into your hands. Imagine that your hands are curious to find out more about the little toe through touching it. We are all born with healing forces in our hands, but by having been forced to use them in a tense and controlled way most of the time, they might have turned into stiff and tense 'robots'.

Think of a blind person who tries to find out about textures and shapes without seeing them. Try to feel the shape of your bones, muscles, tendons and tissue. Sometimes you have to press quite hard to feel something.

Massage your toes with rubbing strokes. You might feel that the area around the knuckles is knotted or tighter then the rest of the toe. Small 'fluid-cushions' might be felt underneath your toes.

Numbness or pain is an alarm sign for you, to spend more time with massage in that area.

Painful or numb areas often indicate, that there is an energy blockage. It can very well be the beginning of arthritis.

Go through massaging all your toes slowly. If you find yourself getting bored or thinking of other things, you might need to press a bit harder to get a response to your massage. Imagine that the feet are like a telephone where you can call different parts of your body.

The answers will be responses such as:
- a deep breath
- a feeling of electrical currents running through the body
- sounds from your intestines, known as peristalsis
- a meditative sensation of emptiness in the head
- burping
- yawning
- wanting to stretch
- sensations in the stomach or belly, similar to those you get before taking a test or meeting someone you are scared of.

Getting some of the above responses will make you more interested in carrying on with the massage. If you should not get any of those responses, do not give up but be patient. You will get them eventually. After having massaged the toes go to your instep.
We tend to tense our muscles and breathe more shallow or stop breathing when we are afraid. This is a simple survival mechanism that creates muscular armour for protection. Thus the muscles of toes, fingers, instep and heals are quite often very tense.
To release the tension, we sometimes have to work quite hard. On the instep it could be a good idea to use a stone for the massage in order to apply a stronger pressure.
After that, work on the Achilles tendon on the back of the heel. Take the muscle and tendon between thumb, middle and index finger and press. Do not forget to breathe with an open mouth. Now compare how this foot feels different from the other one, which you haven't treated yet.

Exercises
There are various exercises you can do to make you feel more grounded. The first: one is called the 'Lowen bow', named after

Alexander Lowen, psychotherapist who worked with the body and used so-called 'bioenergetic' exercises.

Lowen Bow

You are standing with your feet parallel apart, the fists tucked in the back of the waist, legs, knees and pelvis stretched forward, the chest stretched out and the head bent backwards so that your body is forming a bow. You breathe through your open mouth in this very uncomfortable position. The shaking or vibrating of the legs can be a result of this exercise, which you should not do too long at a time.
This position should be followed by an exercise, where you allow your body to bend forwards and hang down loosely, still breathing through the mouth. Slightly bend your knees in this position.
After a while you can touch the floor with your hands and push your buttocks up, whereby the knees will stretch a bit more.
Later move from there into a position similar to the 'dog pose' (yoga exercise), simply walk your hands forwards on the floor. Try to keep your heels closely to the floor. To finish, move further down into a 'squatting position', you can rest your heels on two cushions and fold your hands behind your neck. Try to relax.
Other ways of grounding yourself are dancing, especially free dance without any particular steps, moderate running, walking, cycling and cleaning the floor.
In my practice I use gems, gem and flower essences for lots of different ailments of the body and the mind. You can hold a stone and feel your energy moving straight into your feet. Especially black, brown and silver stones can help you to ground yourself. Using a flower or gem essence can have a deeper and more general effect on the whole body and mind. They can work on your internal organs. Negative states of mind can be balanced and eased.

Gems and gem essences for grounding are:
- Garnet (Hessolite)
- Labradorite
- Black Tourmaline
- Obsidian
- Staurolite
- Jet

Flower essences for grounding are:
- Elm
- Sunflower
- Blackberry

Counselling Exercises
Counselling has always been a very useful tool for finding out more about yourself. Usually nobody will listen to you as long and carefully .If you haven't got a counsellor, use a journal and write things down. The following exercises can be very useful:

Talk or write about the following topics for 10 minutes or more
- Pains, tension and injuries I have had on my feet.
- What kind of shoes or socks have I been wearing? (Material, colour)
- Do I like my feet?
- Imagine that you are talking as one of your feet about the way they feel.

Visualisation Exercise (Inspired by polish healer Lilla Bek)
Lie down on your back in a comfortable position. Make sure that you are warm enough. Close your eyes and breathe for a while through your open mouth. Imagine that the mouth is like an open door, receiving the breath. The throat muscle is relaxed and soft, allowing the breath to enter freely all the way through the neck. Imagine the tunnel of the neck padded with soft velvet. Let the breath then enter

the lungs. Visualize the lungs as upside down trees with many small branches and imagine that the breath is flowing freely and deeply through all the branches. Be passive and receiving, do not force anything to happen. Just relax.

The breath can be like a three-year-old child, who wants to do everything alone, but has to be watched all the time by the mother on its way. Be aware and relax the breathing muscles. Allow the chest to expand sideways. Then let the breath flow back in its own way. Watch your very own rhythm patiently. Do not allow thoughts to interrupt your awareness for too long. Always come back to the breath.

Breathing into the Toes and Legs

This exercise is helpful for going to sleep, relaxing, grounding, energising and warming the feet.

Imagine that you are breathing into the big toe of your right foot. Watch it getting warm and relaxed. Visualise the energy centre starting to move and come to live within the top of the toe as if you were lighting a candle on a Christmas tree.

Then breathe into your next toe and watch it getting warmer and more relaxed. It will probably take a while until your toes will respond to this exercise. Go through all the toes of your right foot. Then imagine that with your in-breath the warmth of your toes is spreading into your whole right foot. Do the same with your left toes and foot. Now you have got two warm feet. Imagine, that with your in-breath, the warmth of your right foot is spreading up the leg to the back of your knee and with your out-breath it moves down from the knee to the toes.

Do the same exercise with your left leg. Then do it with both legs, simultaneously. Imagine that with your in-breath, the warmth of your right foot is spreading up the leg to the buttocks and with your out-breath it is moving down to the toes. Do the same with your left leg, and then do it with both legs. Now you should have two warm legs. This exercise is worth practising, whenever you cannot sleep, it will also help you to relax and think less. Practise it in small steps and eventually you will get results.

Release the Blocked Energy in Your Legs

I came to the belief that foot massage, especially deep massage on the bones of the feet, is the most basic massage we usually need. But once the feet have been massaged properly it is time to concentrate on the other bits of the leg. The toes are the main exits for the energy from the whole body and especially from legs, genitals, belly and lower back.

We often 'walk over our ankle' and thus loose our grounding. We cannot 'stand on our own feet'; we are unable to move with our own individual pace. Kicking mainly with the right leg can express anger and release tension in calves and knees. Often therapists use 'kicking a cushion or having a temper tantrum with both feet while lying on the back with bent knees' for their clients to let off steam from repressed feelings.

If you cycle too fast uphill or run with your calves and knees tensed up you can build up a residue of fluid in the calves, which might block the energy, to flow down the leg. The fluid can cause swellings that are often painful.

Synthetic tights, socks and trousers and pointed shoes or shoes with high heels can hinder the flow of energy. It is important to always dress warmly enough especially around the genitals, the belly and the feet. Cold bums and feet do not allow much blood or energy flow.

The calves can usually contain suppressed anger whereas the thighs hold more resentment and bitterness. I usually warn my clients after I have worked deeply on their thighs or calves that they might get very tired or feel heavy and remember old feelings of frustration from the past.

If we don't express those feelings the suppressed energy can easily attract fluid and settle down in the body as a fluid cushion, muscle tension or calcification around the bones.

If the calves are full of fluid it is important to put them up on a chair to allow the fluid to flow down towards the intestines. Only then the freed energy can move out via the toes.

Visualize the legs as roads with traffic. The knees are situated on the 'arc of the road' and thus get most of the accidents and traffic jams. Therefore we have loads of 'waste products' around the knee. Above the knee, on the inner side and underneath the knee we usually find areas of collected fluid, which needs to be released through massage or dancing.

It is good to sit as much with bent knees as you possibly can preferably on the floor or a hard surface. If you cannot bend your knees any more it is important to slowly work towards it and every day bend them a little more although it might be slightly painful in the beginning. Some slow forms of yoga mostly use exercises to stretch tight muscles and breathe into them. The squatting position (also to be recommended on the toilet) the dog pose and the plough are good ones to start with.

Last year while I was travelling through the south of India for two months on my own I was impressed by the way people were sitting on the floor to attend lectures in the different ashrams.

Even the very old people sat with their knees up and bent – In Europe a position which you can only watch being used by children under eight years old.

I have described the visualization and breathing exercise where we imagine that we are breathing into each toe. This exercise is a basic one for deeply relaxing every part of the leg, allowing the energy to flow more and for helping us to go to sleep, or to release a state of mental tension simply by directing the energy from the head to the toes.

Self-Massage of the Leg

For the massage of calves and thighs it is helpful to lie on a matras or blanket on the floor and put the legs up on a chair. Start with foot massage as described in the first chapter 'Ground your feet'. Then work on the bones around your ankles as if you would polish them thoroughly. The Achilles tendon reaches from the heel to the back of the knee. Take the tendon between thumb and index finger and squeeze it gently. Work your way from the heel up to the back of the knee. The further you go up the more difficult it becomes to touch the tendon. You probably have to work on the fluids instead. Imagine that you are milking a cow then you most likely get results such as fluid-like belly sounds, burping, deep breathing and energy movements along legs and arms.

Never forget to breathe with an open mouth. Massage the big front bone along the calf with a firm rubbing movement. For massage on the knee you should try to sit on the floor with your leg stretched out. Then massage the knee bone by imagining the shape of the knee and add as much pressure as necessary by firmly rubbing the knee with your fingertips.

You'll be surprised how sensitive the knee can become after a few minutes of massage. Quite often pain in the knee can be healed with simple massage. Early arthritis needs a lot of attention. Things that have been settling in over 20 years or more cannot just be rubbed off within a few minutes or days. The massage can sometimes increase the pain before it goes. Inflamed areas should not be massaged but treated with Rescue Cream and healing on the aura. To massage the thigh put your leg back on the chair. The muscle above the instep is usually very tense and needs a firm pressure to let go. Then go to the big muscle on top of the thigh and add enough pressure with the thumb or the knuckles to relax it all the way down to the knee. Then try to work on the muscle outside with your whole hand. The thighs are one of the more difficult places for massage. It is not easy to release the often deep-seated tension in this area. Usually we have to add more pressure than anywhere else and quite often the frustration and anger which might be following can cause disappointment. Finish the massage with strokes down the leg.

Flower essences for the knees
- Isopogon
- Macrocarpa
- Wild Potato Bush
- Californian Poppy

Flower essences for the feet
- Sunshine Wattle
- Bauhinia
- Dog Rose
- Silver Princess
- Bottlebrush

Arms and Heart

Once the energies are flowing freely through our toes, feet and legs we might also start to feel the energy moving through our fingers, hands and arms. This is called the 'Echo-effect. Hands are easier to approach than feet. We can work on them whenever we are waiting for something, for example in the tube, train or in a doctor's waiting room.

Balance the Energies in Your Hands
Polarity

Balancing the energy in the right and left hand and foot, balancing the right and left side of the body will bring you in touch with the idea of polarity. Day and night, sun and moon, male and female, yin and yang are all polarities that exist on earth. The psychologists have created terms such as inner child and inner parent, mind and feeling. The Kahuna, a tribe from Hawaii, used the terms middle and lower self. Rudolf Steiner wrote about Ahriman and Lucifer.

Usually the right side of the body is more connected with terms such as: male, sun, day, yang, inner parent, mind and Ahriman. This side is more active, uses rules, numbers and measures things, whereas the left side is more connected with terms such as: female, moon, night, yin, inner child, feeling and Lucifer. The left side is more passive, spontaneous, and creative and uses more imagination. The two can also be seen like picture frame and picture or like parent and child.

Let us imagine that part of our personality is more like an ' inner parent' whereas the other is more like an 'inner child'. Most of the time we probably act like a parent and are suppressing or controlling the 'inner child'. The 'inner child' will try to control us by making us feel things such as anger or fear. If we choose not to feel things, the 'inner child' can make us ill and thus force us to give it the attention it deserves. The 'inner child' can also make us feel dependent on

things such as money, drugs and food or people.
Different alternative therapies such as Acupuncture, Bach Flower Remedies, Touch for Health, Rebirthing and Biodynamic Psychotherapy (just to name a few) are all using very similar concepts. In psychotherapy the therapist often will try to help their client to strengthen the suppressed 'inner child'. They might do this by helping the client to create a third personality. This personality is neither child nor parent and will help the 'inner child' and the 'inner parent' to find solutions to their problems.
One way to achieve this is conscious listening.
This third personality, sometimes called the Higher Self, dwells in the middle space all along the spine and especially in our heart.

Blockages

What is a blockage? Let's imagine that energy which is flowing freely through body, arms and legs tends to get blocked.
Energy attracts body fluid (lymphatic fluid).
If a child reaches out a hand to take a sweet, energy moves through her arm and hand. If the child is stopped by the parents, through shouting or hitting, this energy cannot move and will attract body fluid.
Fluid and energy will form a blockage, maybe a fluid cushion that will be 'sitting in the tissue' and hinder the rest of the energy from moving. If the blockage is not dissolved, it will solidify and move further inside the body. First it can tense the muscles, later it might crystallize around the bone.
Blocked areas will tend to get painful or numb and the flow of blood and energy will decrease, thus creating a basis for illness and disease. Norwegian Psychotherapist Gerda Boyesen found one way to dissolve energy blockages. She started to use a stethoscope on the stomach. By listening to the sounds of the intestines during massage as a feedback from the body she was able to help the energies to move out through arms and legs. Thus the energy can enable the fluids with the dissolved crystals, lacto acid, adrenalin

and other waste products to find their way out via the intestines. Gerda called this process 'psychoperistalsis' (digestion of emotions). Usually, in a healthy body, the psychoperistalsis will always re-establish itself if it gets out of balance.

On the next pages you will find *The Tina Story*, a short comic which I created for my clients to help them understand the theory of Biodynamic Psychotherapy.

During or after the treatment people can have dreams, and they might remember and express feelings and images that they had suppressed as a child while those energy blockages were developing in their body.

We usually write and do most of our work with our right hand. It is an interesting experience to draw or write with the left hand, carry things on the left shoulder and thus try to create a balance between the right and left side of the body. We usually were told as children how to write or sew or play the piano in the right way. Fear of doing things wrong often created tension in our arms and hands.

Doing something in an enjoyable way will loosen tension and blockages. Creativity can only develop in a space free of any judgment. Thus I often ask people with tense hands and fingers what they enjoy doing with their hands. Sometimes they have to go back to childhood to remember when they enjoyed making figures out of clay or plasticine and baking cakes, finding their own tunes on the piano or putting seeds into the earth.

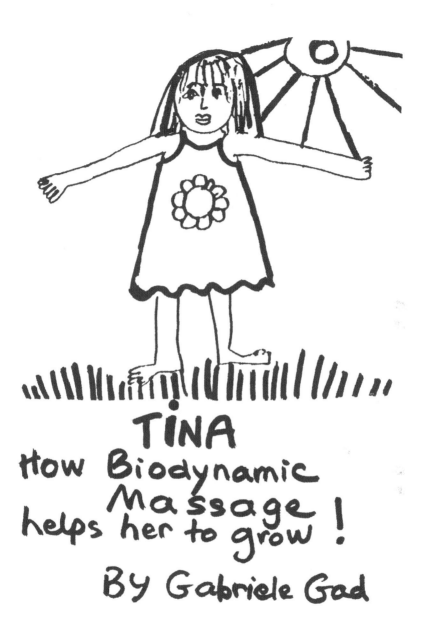

TINA
How Biodynamic Massage helps her to grow!
By Gabriele Gad

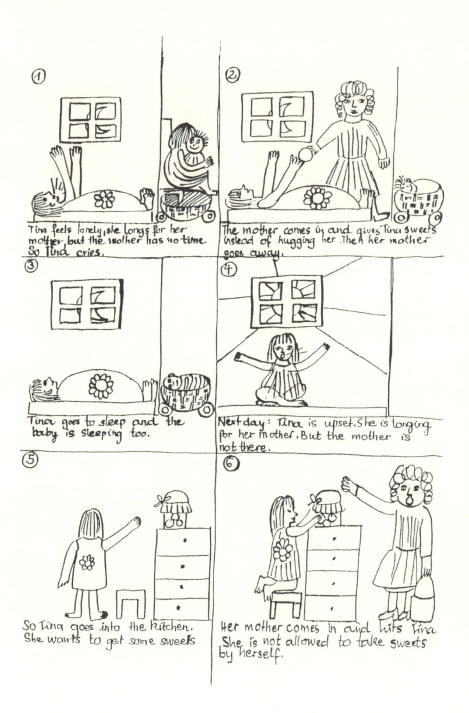

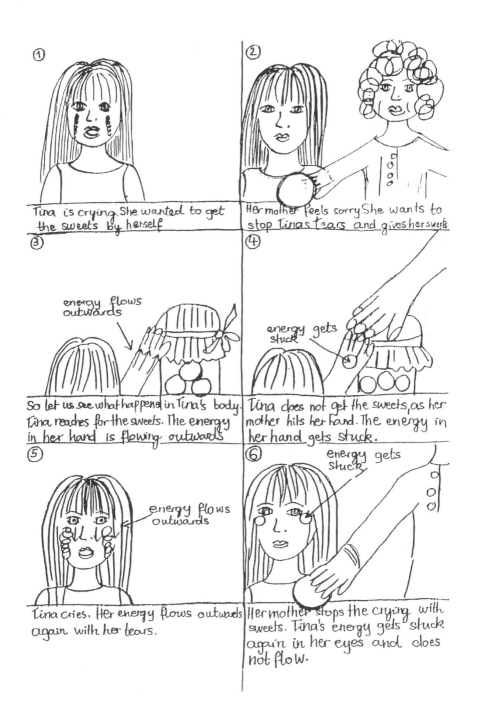

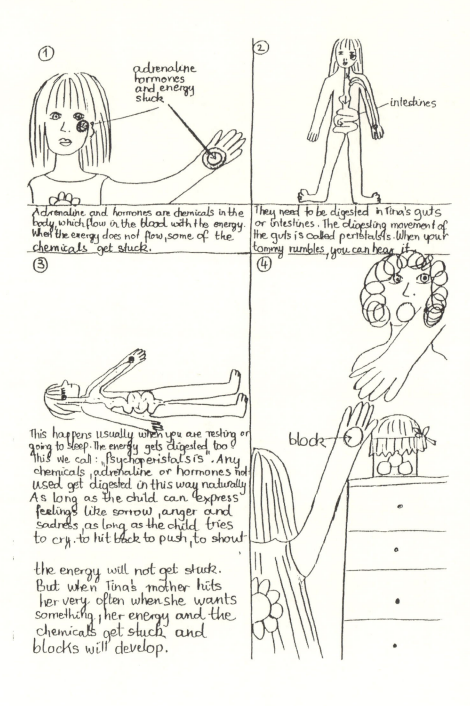

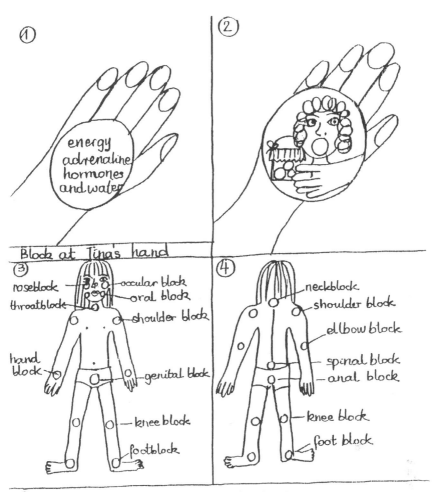

Blocks start to develop all over the body.
The muscles become very tense. The intestines become tense. Digestion problems, back aches, bad posture, stiff neck, tics in the face, overeating, bad eyes, headaches start to develop. When the blocked areas get massaged, the blocks start to dissolve. The body begins to digest the stuck chemicals. The belly begins to rumble. Psychoperistalsis starts working again.

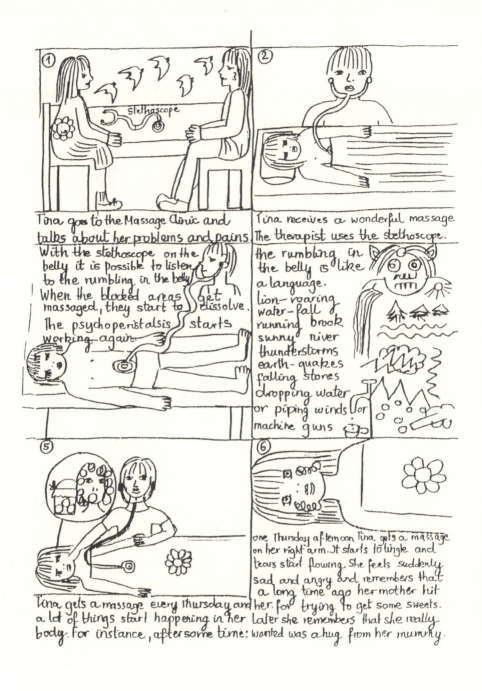

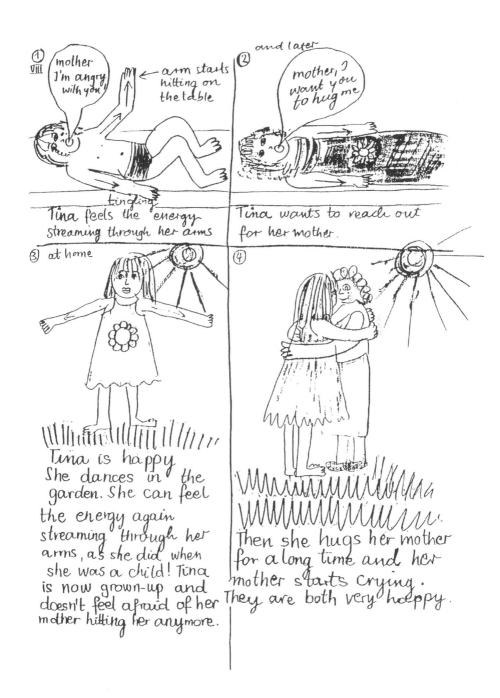

Some information about energy-blocks:

			is forbidden		
👁 eyes	to look at things and people			reaction: child wants to cry child can get short sighted or cross-eyed → eye-block	child must go to sleep at a special time, child must look away, close the eyes
👄 mouth	to talk, sing cry, taste, eat suck, drink, bite or cough			reaction: spitting, vomitting lips get tight throat gets tight throat or → mouth-block, tics jaw-block, tics	child must only drink and eat at a certain time child must keep quiet, or talk to somebody
👂 ears	to listen to sounds			reaction: child doesn't listen anymore — closes his ears ear-block	child must listen to the parents advice listen to the teacher, not listen to music
✋ hands	to touch things and people to hold, feel, embrace, form to suck at the thumb			reaction: child wants to hit back, to push away, to throw away → child "sucks" at cigarettes hand-arm blocks shoulder-neck blocks	child must keep the hands quiet-
🦵 legs	to go away to run to dance to kick			reaction: kicking pelvic-leg-knee and foot blocks stiff legs	child must sit quiet

Hand Massage

Massage of hands and fingers can help you to prevent arthritis, repetitive strain injury and carpal tunnel syndrome.

Find a comfortable space to sit, preferably leaning with your back against the wall. Most of the things that I wrote about foot massage can be applied to hand and finger massage too. We try to breathe with an open mouth. While you massage feel what's underneath, the bone, the muscle and the tendon. Usually the area around the knuckle is blocked and either numb or painful. Fluid cushions occur mostly underneath the lower fingers. On cushions you work with a soft, intuitive rubbing movement.

But the knuckles can be massaged with more pressure. A bone that aches when you are pressing hard is usually already calcified. Crystals of blocked energy are layering the bone. Once you start to rub and breathe you need to watch out for the signals from the body that will tell you, that something is moving.

The Signals from Inside the Body

- A deep breath
- Peristaltic sounds
- Wormlike uncurling movements in the tummy
- Slightly acidic feelings of fear and yearning in the stomach or belly
- Sensations of electric currents running through arms and legs
- A feeling of meditative emptiness in the head
- Burping
- Yawning
- Wanting to stretch

All these signals can be a feedback from inside the body. Sometimes pain might appear or increase and affect the whole surrounding area for a few days before it disappears in the end. In the beginning you might feel rather impatient. But just think how much your hands and fingers have worked for you day by day like servants. Now you can give them some attention for a change as a thank you towards your body.

Once you start feeling the feedback signals from inside the body, you will start to enjoy the massage. Having finished the fingers go to the fluid cushions on your palm. Work especially on bits that are numb or painful. Then concentrate on the prolongation of the finger bones and the tendons and muscles that are attached to them on the top of your hand. Rub them firmly to make them relax. Do not forget to breathe through an open mouth.

The bones of the wrist are the next area you should focus on. Then compare the right hand with the left hand. Does the massaged hand feel any different? It would be very helpful for you to find a friend to work on. You will be surprised how much they will like the massage.

Energy Centres or Chakras

Energy attracts fluid to form a solid unit – the energy blockage. The free life energy is thus imprisoned and cannot move freely anymore. Thus we have less energy for everyday activities.

Through the energy channels, the so-called meridians, energy is moving up and down the body. If energy and fluid are not 'fighting' they can come together in the middle of the body all along the spine and form energy centres, the so-called chakras. Clairvoyants can see those chakras as coloured flowerlike shapes spinning round all along the spine. That's where our third party, the 'higher self,' can settle down and create harmony between the right and left side. When people start to become more aware of themselves and start working towards inner and outer balance and harmony in their life, these chakras will start to open and spin around.

Through those chakras we create invisible links with other people, with past and future experiences and with higher consciousness and spiritual realms.

There are small chakras on the top of our toes and fingers as well. They start spinning round when our hands and feet are feeling vibrant and full of life.

Creative Expression Exercise

Put your favourite slow music on. Then sit down in a comfortable chair and relax. Breathe through your mouth. Your hands are resting on your legs. Imagine that the music is slowly waking up your fingers of the right hand and they begin to move gently, one after the other to the music. Then the hand starts to move about and eventually your whole arm is dancing and moving to the music. After a while the right hand starts to wake up your left hand like the prince of the fairytale 'sleeping beauty' and the two hands are slowly dancing and moving together. They stretch and move upwards and downwards, backwards and sideways. After five or ten minutes let them settle down again slowly. Close your eyes and rest. Breathe and feel your body.

Nowadays so many people develop pain in their hands. Automatic movements as well as tense activities with hands and fingers can cause energy blockages whereas creative expression such as dancing, tai-chi, creative writing, free creative painting, forming sculptures or cakes and the exercise above can help to unblock and free energies and dissolve blockages.

Love from the Heart to the Hands

Once we have worked on our hands and feet as the exits for the energy we can think of them as roads where the traffic can now flow freer to the torso and its organs. The heart is the organ that is usually closely connected with the left arm. The energy wants to move freely from the heart to the hands and from the hands to the heart.

Once the energies in the hands are released, we need to work on blockages in the bones and muscles of the lower and upper arm, the elbow and the shoulder. One of the most relaxing techniques that I know is called 'lifting'. But you will need a partner to practice on.

Lifting

Ask your partner to sit or lie down comfortably. If they lie down, give them a blanket to keep warm. Ask them to breathe through their open mouth if possible and relax. Then start working on their left arm as follows:

Put your right hand under their elbow for support. With your left hand you are gently lifting their hand up. Try to move the arm, bend it carefully in different directions towards the heart, up the head and then down again.

If you can feel any resistance to move in your partners arm, rest a moment and then gently encourage the arm to go along with you. If there is resistance, you can practice the same movement a few times

until your partner starts to let go and trust you a bit more.
For many people it is not easy to allow another person to move their arm.
It sometimes needs a big amount of confidence and concentration to relax the arm and to release old patterns of tension.
If someone has been shocked by an accident, if the arm has been broken or bruised it will take a long time to relax the muscles and tendons.
You will be surprised how relaxed the left arm will be compared to the right one after having worked on it for about five or ten minutes!

The Heart
People who have been brought up with foster parents or in an orphanage, those who lost one or both of their parents in childhood or had to be separated from them early in life usually feel blockages in their chest. The chest might be sunken or they could be suffering from asthma. There are lots of ways blockages could show as illness or disease in early or later stages in their life. Once a child has been abandoned by the parent, especially in early childhood, the energy in the heart tends to 'freeze'. The energy cannot move towards the mother any more and attracts fluid to form a blockage that makes the child feel safe and able to survive. The child withdraws the feelings it had for the parent, especially for the mother. This does not happen without tears and dramatic scenes where the child will do everything to overcome the separation and the feelings of loneliness. But since children usually are small and dependent, there is not much they can do if the parents decide, for example, to send them to a boarding-school at an early age. The separation of the parents in early childhood will always leave severe scars for the child.
Body-orientated psychotherapy can be very helpful for those people. The biodynamic therapist will usually work a lot on the heart and chest to help the frozen energies to be released and move into the

arms. Emotional expression will go together with the treatment. The client can try to talk to their parent by using a cushion. They might cry, and express their anger and sadness for a long time until they can start to forgive them and trust other people as much as they trusted their parents in the very beginning.

This session should preferably be led or accompanied by a therapist.

Self-Massage

Lie down in a comfortable position. Make sure that you are warm. Breathe through your mouth into the upper chest. Then put your right hand on your sternum and breathe into your hand. Watch your breath getting deeper. Then start to massage your sternum. Find the right pressure by watching out for 'responses from the body'(see last chapter). Start to massage your ribs. Painful bones are always an indication for blocked energy. Take plenty of time for your massage. There is space to say things to your parents or friends, although they are not there. Saying things that you feel can unblock your energies, especially if you are saying them in an emotional way. Making sounds is another powerful way of unblocking energies. If you feel the energy in your heart moving, finish the session with gentle strokes from the heart down the arm to the hands. Afterwards allow yourself some leisure time without any pressure.

Flower Essences

Edward Bach, a doctor working in Harleyford Road, was the first one to develop a comprehensive system of flower essences. It took many years for his new medicine to get through to the people. Even nowadays, many people do not know, what flower and gem essences are and how such a cheap and simple tiny bottle of drops could have such a big effect on their lives. There is a wide variety of essences on the market, but for the beginner I would always recommend to start with a thorough study of the Bach Flower Essences. German Psychotherapist Mechthild Schaeffer wrote a book about the use of the essences. I prefer it to Bach's book because it explains the different negative states of mind ever so well. Just by studying the book slowly, you will acquire a thorough understanding of the whole range of those different states of mind, as Dr. Bach has called the various feelings and ways of being entangled by the ego. He has found seven headings for the 38 different remedies that are made by the use of homoeopathic principles. One of the headings is fear. There are remedies for five different forms of fear such as follows:

- Aspen: fear of the unknown, the occult and the future
- Red Chestnut: fear about other people
- Rock Rose: fear that causes bodily sensations, mostly in the solar plexus
- Cherry Plum: fear to loose your head and go mad
- Mimulus: fear of known things, shyness and vulnerability

The scope of Bach Flower Essences seems to include the whole range of negative states of mind, a person can have. You can mix up to six remedies in one 20 ml dropper bottle (one remedy stock bottle is only about £3–7).

If you are really interested in your own personality, there is nothing better you can do, than always asking yourself "how do I feel right now?" and "which remedy would I need right now?"

Holding a stock bottle in your hand can be another way of finding out the remedy you need at a time. Sensitive people can feel sensations in their hand or the rest of the body, when they are holding the right remedy. Sensations range from feelings of warmth, stomach sounds (peristalsis), sensations of electric currents to itchiness.

Tiny tensing movements in the intestines might indicate the start of elimination and thus show the cleansing effect of a particular remedy. Some people prefer working with a pendulum instead. Flower Essences are not just taking fear away. They slowly enable you to learn how to deal with your fear. Other essences help to gain more self-confidence or overcome your feeling of loneliness or impatience. It is quite unique how subtle an essence will work on you – not like a drug where you get the feeling of being hit with a sledgehammer. Some remedies make you feel better straight away; those are the ones to start with. Other remedies can get you into all kinds of strange moods, memories from the past will come up and you quite often need a lot of courage to keep taking the remedy and face the changes. Therapy usually does not heal you straight away. It throws you out of your usual balance into chaos and then you have to work hard to come to a new and better balance. A lot of essences work like that. But not everybody wants to grow, if it is painful. Some people want to leave old negative feelings and experiences under the carpet and choose rather not to look at them. People who have hurt them are excluded from their lives. Although the old grudges are never ever released and only slumber in a distant corner of ourselves, as long as we haven't dealt with them. Dealing with them properly means sometimes going through old memories and feelings again, digesting them, putting them into a new context and, most importantly, forgiving other people and forgiving ourselves again and again. But be careful and always choose the right time for taking your remedy

Bach Flower Essences for the hands and the heart
- Scleranthus for emotional balance and decision making
- Agrimony for personal expression and being able to say 'no' to other people's suggestions
- Gentian for depression and gaining confidence
- Wild Rose for resignation helps to gain new energies
- Honeysuckle and Walnut for loss and letting go with the past.

Gems
Gems for the heart are usually pink, red or green:
- Rose Quartz helps to deal with father figures, missing someone, any emotional upsets
- Aventurine helps children to feel at home
- Jade to develop creativity, especially musical talents.

Putting one of these stones on your heart can help you to go to sleep and balance your feelings.

Spiritual Healing
When I trained at the Boyesen Centre for Biodynamic Massage and Psychotherapy in London, Gerda Boyesen also taught me how to work on the aura. It is not enough to massage the physical body; some people need 'massage' on the auric body as well. My experience is, that slim, subtle, vegetarian, non-smoking and non-drinking women are usually the ones most sensitive to aurawork and Flower and Gem Essences.
The best way to learn aurawork and spiritual healing is to start with your own body.

Exercise
Sit down in a comfortable position preferably on the floor and push your hands together. Breathe through the mouth and imagine, that you are gathering a lot of energy between your palms. Start forming a ball of energy with circular movements of your hands. Let the ball grow to the size of a football and then with both hands spread the fluffy invisible substance round your head, shoulders and chest. Imagine you are dealing with cotton wool to wrap delicate porcelain. Try to find out, where on your body you want to have extra energy. In some places you might already have too much energy. Usually the left side of the body feels more depleted of energy.
Try to move your hands away from the skin like cats do, when they use their paws on your pullover. When you start, to develop sensitivity in your palms you can feel the gluey energy growing under your palms. Once you have caught it, you can slowly enlarge it. Thus a damaged, squashed or depleted aura can be fluffed and repaired similar to the way you shake squashed feather duvets.
Quite often the energy is blocked in the heart. An invisible vortex or auric hole would might then appear above the heart. The technique described above can help blocked energy to be released to a certain

extent. The auric hole can be fixed for a while, the aura repaired. Working with good results on your aura sometimes needs a long time of practice. It is always good to see a healer to explore the sensation of getting healing. You don't have to be ill to ask for healing. Members of the National Federation of Spiritual Healers are working in many places for donations. I am a full member and quite often I use spiritual healing together with biodynamic massage.

So far I have been writing about biodynamic principles around the heart area. Now I will write about the organ itself and its connection with the heart meridian and the heart chakra, the feelings of love and forgiveness versus anger, sounds and colours relating to the heart, its connection with the sun and the pituitary gland. I will also mention gem and flower essences that are good for the heart.
In her book *The (Musical) Fifth is Man*, Felicitas Muche describes the heart as a rhythmical organ in the middle of the body. It seems to be formed out of a spiral movement. The heart is a muscular organ of will. In the Book of Genesis, in the Bible, we read about the paralyzation of God's will, which used to stream through our heart. Our own human will is used through the heart, as our physical will centre. A weakness of muscles brings about a weakness of will. The will can be seen as a balancing act between warmth and fire. The tone of the muscle must be right; it must not be too tight or too loose.
In the human heart organ some of us can hear the double vibration of the third (the third note of a musical scale). In the long and dark tone of the veins they hear the minor and in the small arterial light tone the major third. They can hear one tone after the other.
Cross muscles are usual pointing towards a future expression of the will. We use the will of love to hug people from our heart with our arms and hands. We 'take someone to our heart' or we cling to something with 'all the threads of our heart'.
Man sustains himself in his whole life through the heart forces. As an active organ the heart can form a bridge between the above and the below.

The crown arteries are crowning the heart like a 'crown of thorns'. Auriculae (Latin) means reddish shimmering gold and shows the connection between 'gold' and the heart. Gold also stands for the sun. Someone who has a golden heart can have the whole solar system inside their body.

Like an outer shell of protection the heart and the lungs are surrounded by the rib cage. In the heart we can experience the twofold communication between 'creator and creation'. In St. John's Revelation 2.14 we can read that the angel writes to the community in Thyatira:

> "This says God's son whose eyes are like fire flames and his feet are like a glowing golden heart. All the communities shall see that it is me that examines their kidneys and hearts."

Why should they only mention these two organs? Some people believe that in the next stage of the earth, the so-called Jupiter stage, we won't have any more lungs, liver, spleen, brain, genitals and no metabolism. The heart however will remain our central organ. The throat will work as our future reproductive organ of the word, the kidneys as an organ of divine wisdom will replace the thinking from the brain.

The Heart Chakra

The heart chakra is supposed to be formed out of 12 lotus leaves, the seat of the 'voice of silence'. Here all divine things are revealed through the inner word. To fully control the 12 leaved lotus, we have to be able to be in full control of all our thinking.

The wider the heart chakra is open, the more we will be able to love unconditionally. From here we form chords to the heart chakras from the people we love. One speaks of 'heart strings'. An open-heart chakra often brings tears of compassion into our eyes.

People whose heart chakra spins clockwise usually manage to create good things in their lives and they can see others supporting them and their tasks wherever they do. Their will is in agreement with God's will.

With people whose chakra spins anticlockwise the opposite is true. They think that God's will and the will of others are opposed to their own will and that the others will always create obstacles to get in their way. These people function by control and they seem to make their lives safe by controlling others.

Exercise for Strengthening the Heart:
Stand with both arms stretched out as if they would surround a golden ball in front of your heart. Breathe through your nose and feel the chi in your hands increasing. Do the exercise for about ten minutes to start with.

The Heart Meridian

The Heart Meridian is 'yin' (yin- female, yang -male) and the feelings related to this meridian are anger versus love and forgiveness. (angk = to choke, to oppress, angina pectoris, anger – to strangle). The outer meridian starts under the arm and goes from there at the inner side of the arm towards the inner angle of the nail of our little finger. The inner meridian goes from the heart sideways across the chest towards the arm. Another branch goes through the diaphragm towards the small intestine, a third branch goes through the neck and face up to the eyeball.

Physical indications are:
Dryness of the throat, strong thirst, pain in chest and ribs, nervous heart beat, bladder problems, urination problems and bad sight Restlessness, nervousness, over-sensitivity, hysteria, sudden mood changes, too much laughing, depression, sleeping problems, disinterest, lack of courage, forgetfulness, pressure to keep sighing, over-expectation, fear of tests, too much talking, anxiety before a performance.
The element fire belongs to this meridian. It relates to warmth energy and to the summer. The taste is bitter, that means bitter food can have an effect on this meridian. Too much joy can have a bad

influence on the heart, for example cause a heart attack.
John W. Garvy wrote a very interesting booklet on the five phases of food relating to the five elements. If there is a deficiency of fire energy you are supposed to eat the following food:
Corn, popcorn, red lentils, asparagus, brussels sprouts, chives, endive, okra, scallions, tomatoes, apricots, guava, raspberry, strawberry.
If there is an excess of fire energy then the following food should be eaten:
Buckwheat, black soybean, aduki bean, kidney bean, sea wheat,, burdock, mushrooms, water chestnut, blackberry, blueberry, cranberry, watermelon.
Red is the colour of the heart-circulation system. Very red skin can thus be an indication for heart-circulation imbalances. At the beginning of high blood pressure the skin vessels can be widened. A very red face of a patient can thus be an important diagnostic sign.
If the heart is disturbed, we should think of a few important issues: Am I having enough time and space in my life to look at my feelings and express them? Is my life rhythmical or do I push everything into an artificial schedule? Are my heart and my head, my feeling and my thinking working harmoniously together? Do I love or live half-heartedly? Do I listen to what my heart is telling me?
The rhythm of our heart is less open to our influence then the rhythm of the breath. If we experience problems with the heart rhythm it could mean an interruption of our deeper order in life. Or it could be an indication that we are too rigid and do not allow ourselves to be carried away with emotions.
Angina pectoris occurs when the blood vessels are hardened and shrunk so that we do not get enough food any more. It means that the heart has become too tight. Thus it needs nitro-glycerine capsules to 'explode' and widen it again.
The heart chakra can be trapped between overactive centres. If the mind is always busy, our solar plexus gets overcharged. Too much food and drugs will overcharge the abdomen. If we talk too much

influencing business talk, the throat chakra gets too fast. All this can have a weakening effect on the heart muscle.

If we 'fall in love' we are trying to balance our energies. We always attract the ener–gies that we haven't got to make us 'whole'.

Making Love is the Balancing of the Chakras

Our understanding of others is linked to our relationship with ourselves. If we are able to forgive the ones who were close to us then we can really grow spiritually.

In order to love unconditionally we have to be able to overcome our anger first. A lot of people are not even aware of their anger. It comes out in illness and tension and it often shows in their language being over-critical and thus keeping things at a distance.

In therapy I usually encourage people to say the things they do not like first and to accept feelings of resentment, bitterness, envy, jealousy and anger more and more. There is a safe space where they can allow themselves to express feelings without hurting someone. Acting out through role-play and cushion bashing can be a freeing experience.

After having started to accept anger and hate the real love and forgiveness can enter us naturally. First they show in very small signs only and it is good then to be ever so patient and not pushy at all. Otherwise we would only chase them away again.

To finish a session you can use an affirmation for forgiveness.

You could write on one page of a book "I forgive X for…" and on the opposite page the feelings that come up (for example "I could never ever forgive this person as long as I live.") Then go on writing the affirmation of forgiveness for all the people you remember that you are still cross with.

Sometimes you can be lucky and be brought together again with the people you haven't yet forgiven. There is a karmic attraction, I suppose. Once we are dead it is too late to forgive and we then sometimes have to carry these bad feelings around with us for a long time. There are things that we can only accomplish on the earth plane while we are alive. A lot of dead people are actually desperately waiting to be born and fulfil their tasks.

That's why suicide can be a very disappointing experience and not at all as people imagine it to be. They expect it to be peaceful and freeing but the opposite is true. In the beginning it is probably much more confusing and limiting for them then life has ever been before.

A good way to calm our heart is chanting the 'aum' for the heart chakra, which unites our hearts with all the other hearts in oneness. A nice color such as golden or pink (like a Rose Quartz) can be visualized in the heart and give us peace and tranquillity.

Rudolf Steiner in his book *How to Gain Knowledge from the Higher Worlds* describes the heart chakra as a soul organ or lotus flower with 12 petals. Six petals have already been used in the past and the other six have to be developed in this life. Every petal is linked with one quality. The first two petals with continuity and control of thinking arid acting, the third one with the development of duration, the fourth one with tolerance towards beings and objects, the fifth one with belief and trust, the sixth one with a balance in life and feelings.

Some people have linked the heart with the pituitary gland.

The Pituitary Gland

This endocrine gland, which is not bigger than a pea, is situated at the base of the brain. It is a so-called 'ductless' gland (which means the secretions are not gathered in a duct or tube but are passed directly into the blood.) The hormones of the pituitary gland are called Antuitrin, Pituitrin and ACTH. The pituitary affects the uterus muscles, the small blood vessels, kidneys and mostly-female sex organs and it can have an influence on human growth.

Together with the pineal gland, the pituitary forms a gateway to the second nervous system. They can both be described as vibratory rates able to link up with the 'higher self'. The pituitary functions better in the darkness. The pituitary if stimulated by excessive judgment or criticism can restart growth of certain anatomical features such as the nose in middle or later life.

Qualities that can lead to poor functioning of the pituitary and can result in loss of memory and weakening of the intellect are: Excessive judgment and criticism, aloofness, withdrawal, cautiousness about accepting things, pettiness, nitpicking and scepticism.

An old friend of mind used to sing songs to his pituitary gland.

Flower and Gem Essences for the Pituitary Gland
Californian Flower Essences and others:
Almond, Amaranthus, Ginseng, Hops, Koenigin von Daenemark, Papaya, Passionflower, Banana, Californian Poppy, Mallow, Mango, Pennyroyal, Green Rose, Pimpernell, Skullcap, Yerba Mate. Australian Flower Essence: Yellow Cowslip Orchid Gem Essences: Gold, Jasper Picture, Lalis Lazuli, Malachite, Lazurite, Moonstone, Opal, Zirkon, Amethyst, Silver, Ruby, Clear Quartz.

Flower and Gem Essences for the Heart
Australian Flower Essences:
Bluebell, Black-eyed Susan, Red Helmet, Old man baksia, Little Flannel Flower for seriousness in children, grimness in adults.

Californian and other Flower Essences:
Blackberry, Bleeding Heart, Centuary Agave, Cosmos, Comfrey, Honeysuckle, Lotus, Pimpernel.

Gem Essences:
Copper, Emerald, Garnet, Gold, Magnesium, Malachite, Ruby, Rose Quartz, Star Sapphire, Black and Green Tourmaline.

After having worked on the feet, hands, arms and heart we come to an important part of our journey towards the sacrum. We come to our neck and shoulders.

The Neck and Shoulders

After having explored the arms and hands and their link with heart and chest we will dedicate one chapter to the area of our body that is getting most of the tension: our neck and shoulders. Working on computers, typewriters, telephone, watching television, driving, playing the piano or the violin, the flute, the saxophone and the clarinet are just some of the activities that often have a tensing effect on our neck and shoulders.

Release the Tension in Shoulders and Neck

The front of the neck, the area of breathing and swallowing is just as important as the back. Often clients complain about a blockage in their throat. They feel as if they have swallowed an object, their voice tends to be too high or husky, they keep coughing without a cold. The back and the front of the neck work together as a team just like man and woman whereas the front is symbolizing the open receiving part connected with the mouth and the back of the neck stands more for the male supporting and strengthening part. The neck is the link between the head and the body. Breath, food, energy and fluids have to pass through the passage of the neck upwards and downwards. When the neck muscles and tendons are tense, when the vertebrae are calcified and stiff, the passage can easily be blocked. The results can be bad posture, breathing problems, chest problems and many other symptoms. Tension and pain in back, neck and shoulders are a symptom of our present generation.

The spine consisting of 24 free and five cross vertebrae is usually very elastic and flexible. In between the vertebrae are 23 discs, which tend to get worn out. But usually this is not due to over-use, as it might happen to people who lift heavy things and work hard with their body. It is mostly due to under-use and to one-sided use and happens to office workers, drivers and people who do not move enough.

Parts of the body that are not being used enough can disintegrate. In southern countries where people still carry heavy loads on top of their heads there are fewer complaints about aches and pains in neck and shoulders and the people have beautiful postures.

Simeon Pressel in his book *Movement is Healing* thinks that healing of the stiff, sore or tense muscle can only work if the movement is done in a joyful way. The word muscle stems from Latin 'muscalus' which means 'small mouse'. A small mouse is a very lively animal. Children move out of joy. Unfortunately the child's stream of joy is often interrupted far too early.

Why do we feel so touched when we watch the waves of the sea, a waterfall or a river? Does this rich stream of movement have an effect on our stream of movement inside? Many people get excited when they are watching sports. But watching can only give you a glimpse of your own joy to move your body.

It cannot stop the decay of the muscles and limbs and we all seem to go towards this decay since machines have taken over nearly every movement we used to do with our body.

The decay starts with disinterest in movement. Then it grows from a resistance to move into a disability to move. For our metabolism movement is the motor that keeps everything going. If we do not move enough we collect fat and water in our body, which will block further movement.

It then becomes a vicious circle. When too much tiredness and weakness of will overflood the individual they only want to be moved by outside influences.

Sometimes illnesses such as catarrh and fever can soften the muscle tension. Pressel recommends warmth and massage, healing baths, movement exercises, healing eurhythmy and chiropractics.

F. M. Alexander, founder of the well known Alexander Techniques discovered that if the head was sitting on the neck in the right way and with every movement was held in the right proportion to the neck we would have the easiest and healthiest life. When we stand straight the neck should be carried effortlessly and rest in a balanced way on the uppermost vertebra of the neck, and the arms, hands and fingers should hang freely and relaxed.

It all starts with the beginning of school where children are quite often forced to sit still.

They also carry heavy bookcases on one shoulder or one side of their back. The worst happens though when they start writing. They write with a bent back and head, their shoulders come up and they stiffen their fingers around the pen.

Alexander describes how all the different ways of bending the head can affect the posture and have a bad effect on our body – especially on the way we breathe, the function of different glands, the tension of muscles, the deformation of our bones and last, but not least, the way we feel.

The pressure points for a stiff neck are situated in the front of the shoulder above the collar bone, opposite the elbow and 5cm deeper on the side of the elbow, on the root of the big toe and on the little finger 2mm away from the edge of the nail. If you are pressing the right point you should usually feel a slight pain.

Australian Flower Remedies for the neck are:
- Isopogon for poor memory, senility, a controlling and manipulating personality
- Crowea for continuous worrying, feeling not quite right
- Kangaroo Paw for insecurity, lack of awareness and clumsiness

Australian Flower Remedies for the shoulders are:
- Paw Paw for feeling overwhelmed, unable to resolve problems, burdened by decision making
- Dog Rose for apprehension with other people, fearfulness, insecurity and shyness
- Sunshine Wattle for people who are stuck in the past and are expecting a grim future.

Gem Stones and Essences for tension in neck, atlas bone and shoulders are:
- Aquamarine
- Kunzite
- Loadstone
- Magnetite Diamond

Bits of loadstone or magnetite should be placed on the back of the neck from 30 minutes up to three hours. This will stimulate the magnetic or cerebrospinal fluid.

Massage of Neck and Shoulders

In order to massage your own neck and shoulders it is good to lie down comfortably on your back and cover yourself with a blanket. Place a small cushion under your head.

Go to the shoulder muscle, grab it with your whole hand and hold it for a while. Dig with your fingertips deeply into the space underneath on the back. You might even be able to reach with your fingertips a bit further down the back where the 'ego point' is situated just under the shoulder-bone where two layers of muscles are crossing. If you can find the right spot you might feel a sensation going all the way down your arm like electricity.

Do not stop breathing.

Now go back to your shoulder muscle and dig in with the fingertips. Keep massaging the muscle with your whole hand until it feels more relaxed. Massage the area with your knuckles, then do the other side.

In the beginning you might just explore every bit of your body. Try to remember the grade of tension for the future and then gradually form a kind of relationship with the muscle, the bone and the tissue. Once this relationship is strong you will not only feel from inside when the area needs massage but also start to massage it as naturally as you are breathing.

Being massaged on neck and shoulders is of course much better then doing it to yourself.

If you are giving the massage to another person, the use of a table is of a big advantage. You can massage the neck and shoulder from both sides but I prefer people lying on their backs while I sit behind their head on a high chair. I usually begin the massage with laying both my hands symmetrically on the upper chest and wait until they start breathing into the palms of my hands. Then I massage one shoulder as described above. After doing the second shoulder I go to the neck, including the ears and the space behind the ears (see the chapter *Listen to the Waves*.)

In the end I always make strokes from the neck, ears and forehead towards the skull and gently pull the head with the hair towards me. This movement is very soothing and helps to remove stuck energy from the hair and its roots.

Neck and shoulder massage can be followed by massage of the forehead or/and arm and hand massage. It is usually very relaxing and will help people to go to sleep.

Exercises for Neck and Shoulders:

Sit down on a chair. Gently move your head from one to the other side and then move it in a circle always breathing through the open mouth. Afterwards move it up and down a few times. Lift both shoulders up and keep them up for a few seconds. Repeat this movement. Then circle the shoulders backwards and forwards. Stretch your elbows out to both sides while your stretched fingers are touching in front of your chest. Make small circles with your elbows in both directions. Stretch both your arms upwards in all directions and yawn. Do not forget to stretch them backwards as well.

Then inter-link your fingers behind the neck and move the elbows backwards. That will open chest and rib-cage.

Now lie down on your right side with lots of space around you. Put your bent legs on the right side. Try to touch the floor with the left knee. In slow motion make a huge circle with one arm stretching it all the time. Stay a bit longer in the 'tense' areas and gently breathe through your mouth. Then lie on your left side and do the other arm. This position is called 'cosmic man'.

Then lie down on your back to finish with a breathing meditation. Make sure you are warm enough. Close your eyes and breathe through the mouth visualizing the breath as a blue stream of air entering your mouth, passing the neck, entering and widening the lung chest space and then moving back out.

Try to be passive and let the movement of the breath happen to you. Do not force it. Try not to get lost in thinking of other things. Really concentrate on watching the breathing all the time and allowing it to expand in its own slow way.

Then imagine that you are breathing into the thumb of your right hand as if you would light a candle. Imagine that the thumb gets warm and relaxed and the chakra in the finger comes to life. Then breathe into the index finger of the right hand. Go through all the fingers of the right hand slowly. Watch them getting warm and alive. Then repeat the whole sequence with the left hand. Then breathe into both hands simultaneously. Imagine the warmth streaming from the fingers towards the wrist thus warming the whole hand with your breath.

Now imagine that the warmth is spreading with your in-breath from your hand to the elbow and with your out-breath back down to the fingertips. Do one arm after the other and then both arms together. The next breath moves the warmth all the way up from the hands to the shoulders and down again with the out-breath. Take your time with this exercise until you can really feel the warm stream moving inside your fingers and arms. Once you are able to warm both hands simultaneously let the warmth move into the shoulder and then towards your neck.

This exercise needs to be practised regularly and lovingly in very small steps. Once you can feel the warmth moving you will notice the energy stream going away from the head into your arms and out through your fingertips helping you to stop thinking, relax, heal pain and go to sleep. You can then start practising in every position and thus relax at work, at the dentist or during a long office meeting. Our body wants attention especially in the areas that are out of balance. If we give this attention to the body as we would give it to a small child the body will be happy and work for us without 'moaning and groaning'.

The Head

Our journey towards the sacrum has led us from the limbs via the heart towards the head. The first things we usually see are the eyes of the other person.

The Eyes: The Windows of the Soul

Can we trust their eyes? Are they openly looking at us? Are they staring? Or do they seem to think of something else? The eyes seem to be like windows out to the world. Every day we are looking with different eyes. On Monday morning we see the stains on the carpet, the scratches on the furniture and the dirty windows, on Tuesday the lilac of the carpet matching with the mauve of the curtains creating a picturesque contrast to the white cherry blooms outside our bedroom window, gently moved by the wind. Every day we are in a different mood and the mood will have an influence on the way we are seeing things.

Once children start to wear glasses, it does not only mean that their eyes are bad. It often means much more than that. They might be depressed, withdrawn or full of resignation. Their eyes do not want to look at things any more. There is less fun in looking at the world. The eyes withdraw just as if they were making a statement: "I have already had enough of this life, I don't want to see clearly any more." What a lot of sadness lies in this statement! But nevertheless parents and teachers usually ignore those signs. They fit the child forcefully into whatever conditions they have chosen for them. 'You have to fit in, do not even ask why' they seem to say to the eyes of the child. And the child has no choice.

People who had to wear glasses from an early age onwards are usually more critical and more depressed than others. Of course, the body chooses different ways to withdraw. Some children get fat, others get too slim, and others develop asthma or eczema.

It is quite interesting to watch yourself looking at things with different eyes every day and thus study your own moods, feelings and thoughts. But if you are used to pushing yourself the way it was done at school or by parents then you won't be very interested in your 'inner child'.

It is old fashioned to work with pushing and punishment within your own system and it's got to collapse one day and make you ill. This should teach you to be more careful.

So why not start with the eyes? Especially before buying the first set of glasses you should give yourself or your child a chance to find out why the eyes want to withdraw. Bates developed a wonderful system of exercises to improve the eyesight. Since he died, lots of other good books have been written about the improvement of eyesight.

As I am sitting here at the computer typing this article I am wearing a set of pinhole glasses[2] to protect my eyes. Apart from that, I have fixed a small light to help me see the letters more clearly while I am typing.

Twenty years ago I was told to wear glasses. I bought them and only wore them a few times. I didn't like wearing them because my eyes were blurred afterwards and felt hypersensitive. Then I lost them. I am still not wearing any glasses but I carry a magnifying glass with me for important small print. I am still able to read the Evening Standard crossword in the day light. Fortunately I am not in a profession where I am forced to read a lot. Thus I can take things slowly and read whenever I like.

I have started to do various exercises and they seem to have helped me, together with lots of other growth work, to keep my sight in a good state.

Yesterday I saw a television programme about Michael Tippet. He did not wear glasses at 85 years old. And you could see that he was enjoying his work to the full.

---

[2] Pinhole glasses are have opaque lenses with lots of small pinholes that you can focus your eyesight through. *http://en.wikipedia.org/wiki/Pinhole_glasses*

What can you do for your eyes? There is a whole range of flower and gem essences that can help your eyesight to improve.

Flower Essences:
- Star of Bethlehem for shock
- Hornbeam and Eyebright for better vision
- Mustard and Gentian for depressed eyes
- Beech for critical eyes
- White Chestnut for concentration
- Cerato for the balance of the third eye
- Lemon

Gem Essences

These stones can always be used directly on top of the eyelids or held on the aura above the eyes, and the essence can be sprayed or taken internally:
- Citrine for concentration
- Emerald, Malachite, Topaz, Amethyst, Beryl, Clear Quartz and Apophyllite to improve the eyesight

Whilst writing this chapter I have taken breaks to do the first eye relaxation exercise. New age therapist Meir Schneider was almost blind and healed himself with these exercises. He has written some good books about it.

1. I lie down with my back on the floor. My hands are covering both my eyes. The fingers of both hands are lying on top of each other. This is a Bates exercise and it is called 'Palming'. It can also be done in a sitting position.
2. In the morning I usually splash cold and lukewarm water on my eyes – 25 times cold, 25 times warm, 25 times cold.
3. Sometimes I throw a small ball on the wall and catch it with alternating hands. That's the third exercise. It will improve the right left coordination of the eyes.

Then I try to blink a lot and breathe deeply. I avoid neon light and smoky rooms as much as possible.

At the Body, Mind and Spirit Exhibition they sell Pinhole Glasses. These are glasses that can improve your eyesight. You wear them 15 minutes or so per day.

Massage of Forehead, Eyes and Neck

Lie down in a comfortable position. Massage your forehead with your fingertips starting in the middle of the forehead with small strokes towards the temples.

Above your eyebrows are muscles that are usually very tense. I call them the guardians of the eyes. They protect the eye. But if you go through a period of severe tension or trauma, these muscles tense and leave the eye exposed. Then the eye has to withdraw if it does not like the scenery. That's when eye problems usually start.

Therefore it is good to ask what has happened whenever a child starts to wear glasses for the first time. Sometimes a grand parent has died and the child can see the dead person clairvoyantly. But when the child tells its parents they usually say to the child that it's vision is wrong. Then the child's 'third eye' consequently closes and the child is prescribed glasses.

Massage this muscle on top of the middle of the eyebrow with a hard pressure and thus try to relieve the spasm and encourage the muscle to let go and relax. Breathe through your open mouth. Watch out for the signs from the body. Then massage the eyebrows on top and underneath, especially in the corners of the eyes. Feel the bones and try with a 'cleaning' movement to loosen crystals and fluid cushions. Massage under the eye. Tears that haven't been expressed usually settle down under the eye and solidify to 'fluid cushions'

The area under the ears can be pressed hard. Behind the ears you find lots of blocked energy. Fear usually hits us from the back. Guilt can settle down behind the ear and cause ear problems. Massage the bones firmly. Then go to the neck.

Massage all the vertebrae with a cleaning movement. Sometimes it will take a long time to feel some response from within the body. There is even a connection between the bone at the base of the neck and the genitals. After a few minutes work you might feel the lower back starting to relax. Muscular strings right and left from the spine can be 'plucked' with a firm movement like a guitar string. All that helps the energy to move better from the head to the body and arms.

Behind the ears slightly upwards you will find plenty of fluid cushions. They can be pressed hard just on places where they ache and sometimes they burst with an explosive sound. That means that the energy and fluids, which have moved upwards through stress and got stuck, will move down again. Those areas are very much connected with our eyes. Often stiff neck and shoulders and bad eyesight go closely together. Nowadays on-site-massage enables computer stressed office-workers to get a treatment right in the office. I know that modern businesses pay for this service.

Eyes like sunshine, warmth and bright colours, especially yellow and orange, which are vitalising colours for the eye. Eating fruit such as apricots, mangoes, papaya, peaches and vegetables like carrots, pumpkin and squash can have a beneficial effect for your eyesight. They all contain vitamin A. You can buy capsules with the herb eyebright and vitamin A. You can also bathe your eyes in eyebright tea, especially when they feel painful and tired. Black or camomile teabags or cotton wool patches soaked in warm milk will have a soothing effect on the eye as well.

At the Body, Mind and Spirit exhibition I recently had to work on a stall. My eyes were aching because I had not slept enough. I tested a set of glasses with small pads around the eye and a battery. With gentle vibrations the pads were massaging the acupuncture points around my eyes. I must say that it tickled a lot, but that was part of the healing process. The pain in my eyes had gone and I bought a set of those glasses straight away.

Meir Schneider was running an eye workshop at the festival. He made everybody run down the stairs out onto the street and look with closed eyes at the sun, gently turning the neck from one side to the other. This is a Bates exercise and is called sunning. If the sun is not shining, you can use a 100-watt bulb instead to look at. 5 to 10 minutes a day is enough.

Often I get clients who have sleeping problems. Either they cannot go to sleep in the evening or they wake up at three or four o'clock in the morning.

For some people not sleeping means worrying, arguing inside the head, feeling guilty or too excited about things. Thus counselling and psychotherapy in itself would be helpful for them.

Flower Essences for the calming of the mind:
- White Chestnut for ongoing thoughts
- Clematis for 'dreamers'
- Rock Rose for emotional fear
- Gentian for belief
- Pine for guilt.

Gems

Gems can be put on the forehead, the third eye or the heart. Good stones for the forehead are:
- Beryl
- Apophyllite
- Amethyst
- Topaz.

People who never remember their dreams are often quite sad about it. The dream life seems to be a different life we are leading altogether. Stone and flower essences for remembering dreams are:
- Orchid
- Mugwort
- Azurite Malachite.
- Amethyst

It is a good idea to start treating all the different parts of your body like children who are helping you to get on with your life. They want to be looked after, get attention, care, understanding and love, especially if they are not working well.

In these chapters I am trying to give you many ideas how to look after your body, mind and spirit. But the main work has to be done by you.

The Ears: Listening to the Waves

Sometimes I work as a note-taker for deaf students at universities or colleges.

At the City Lit Institute for Adult Education I did a five day training for note-taking and I have learned a lot about the ear, hearing and how to work with deaf students.

It is easy to understand why some of my students tend to get frustrated or irritable about their inability to hear and to be heard. When I was working with a young man who was studying music, I could see it on his face how much he was struggling to hear the different instruments while we were studying the score.

My grandfather was getting deaf in his eighties. My mother used an ear trumpet to make him understand her, but quite often he used to laugh and shrug with his shoulders and that was it. He just did what he wanted.

The ear has the shape of a baby in the womb. Thus you can easily imagine where all the pressure points are located.

I still remember that I used to lie down with my two sons when they were small and twiddle both their ear lobes. Thus they went to sleep in no time.

Ear-acupuncture is often used for cleansing.

Massage on the ear can have a similar effect. Behind the ears we often find blockages on the bones, fluid-cushions or hardened painful bone- areas.

Here at the so-called 'Psychotic wings' where trapped energy can be released to go down to the toes. Thus guilt-feelings can be eased. Emotional balance is affected by the ears and the fluid inside the middle ear. Ear-massage and aurawork on the ear can help with grounding the body.

Recently I attended a workshop with Gerda Boyesen in London. She mostly told us how to draw the 'superego' out of people's ears in the form of short and long spirals (see aurawork) We were working in pairs and the treatment seemed to have a deep effect on most of us. In the passage about spiritual healing on the head I have described how you can draw spirals out of both ears with the in breath and hold them with the out breath. You can draw a second time and then imagine that you are throwing the end of the spiral into the sea. That can have an effect of deep relief and relaxation.

Thorwald Detlefsen in his book about diseases and their underlying emotions relates the faculty of hearing to being passive and obedient. He thinks that hearing problems usually develop in children when they do not want to hear or in old age when we become more rigid and inflexible. Questions such as
'When do I want to listen or not?' and
'To whom do I want to listen?' should be raised and
'Are the poles eccentricity and humbleness in balance?'
Polish clairvoyant Lilla Bek in her book *To the Light* writes about different chakras. The throat chakra is related to the ears. When people began to use the left side of their brains they slowly lost the faculty to see auras, nature spirits and to hear nature's subtle musical sounds such as the music of the stars and the sounds of plants, trees and flowers.

Some sounds can bring our ears up and back. In early times, we could manipulate our psyche through the movement of our ears but today there is hardly anybody left who can move their ears at all. In his book *Healing Sounds: The Power of Harmonics,* Jonathan Goldman writes that our way of listening and our consciousness can be changed by listening to harmonics. He describes hearing as an active experience.

Alfred Tomatoes, French physician, distinguishes between sounds that tire the listener and those that charge the listener. He found that sounds that contain high frequency harmonics (particularly those found in Gregorian chants) are very beneficial to listen to. After the Second Vatican Council, the abbot of a Benedictine monastery felt that the everyday chanting of the monks was not serving any particular purpose. Thus he asked them to stop it. After a while the monks became tired and depressed. The monks were then following a vegetarian diet. A doctor was consulted who put them on a meat and potato diet which only made them much worse. When Dr. Tomatis was called, he asked them to go back to their chanting and immediately they recovered again.

Dr. Tomatis explains that the sound of chanting is not produced in our mouth but in the bones:

> *"It is all the bones of the body singing and it is like a vibrator exciting the walls of the church which also sing."*

Dr Tomatis only needs four hours of sleep per night. By listening to sounds that are rich in high harmonics he charges himself with energy.

Nowadays more and more people are suffering from hearing a constant high-pitched noise (tinnitis.) Stimulating acupressure points can help in the beginning to ease these symptoms. The acupressure points are situated on the inner end of every eyebrow, on top, middle and bottom of the beginning line of the ears and all along the outer earlobe and ear. Press for about 1 to 3 minutes, then release the pressure.

Flower Essences
- Centuary Agave for extensive stress from hearing or memory loss and strengthening of the inner ear canal
- Californian Poppy for middle ear problems affecting the balance, Mallow for loss of hearing in older age.

Australian Flower Essences
- Kangaroo Paw can help unaware, insensitive or clumsy people to increase their sensitivity
- Bush Gardenia improves aural awareness and increases interest in other people and the will to listen to them attentively.

Gems and their essences:
- Picture Agate
- Copper
- Diamond
- Gold
- Kunzite
- Silver
- Amber
- Ruby
- Platinum, Onyx and Rhodonite are all stones that help with hearing and ear problems.

Rhodonite was used in Lemuria to develop our language. At first it helped people to produce mantras, which later became the basis for developing words and sentences. Rhodonite essence can strengthen the inner ear and the bone tissue. It eases ear inflammations.
In his book *Life Energy,* John Diamond describes how every meridian in the body is linked to a particular organ and related to a specific negative emotion and its positive counterpart. The kidney meridian rules the kidneys, eyes and ears and is related to sexual indecision versus sexual security. Thus people who are not sure about their choice of partner might unbalance their kidney meridian and weaken their kidneys, eyes and ears.

The Mouth
We Are What We Eat
Two of the reasons why our spine can get weakened and deformed are: A heavy baby in the womb and overeating. Once the spine is

curved because of the heavy pull that had been applied by a baby or a big stomach, the sensitivity in the curved area might first increase and later decrease. Pain or later numbness can be the result. The nice sensations, the supportive feeling can disappear. Pain is a warning signal and people usually react to it.

But numbness is something we don't feel anymore. And that can be very sad indeed.

So what are the general reasons for overeating? A premature birth? Being fed too much as a baby? Depression and frustration?

One way of eating consciously is starting to follow a macrobiotic diet. Seventeen years ago I came to London. I studied at the Gerda Boyesen Centre for Biodynamic Psychotherapy and I was introduced to Macrobiotic Cooking. I had a boyfriend who worked at the East West Centre and spoilt me with macrobiotic food. In the beginning I did not eat it. But he cooked lots of delicacies to make me interested in macrobiotics. Since that time I always come back to it when I need to.

The macrobiotic style of cooking is based on balancing the meals according to the yin and yang qualities of the ingredients.

Some ways to treat food will make it more yang or yin. Yin plums get more yang when kept in salt for one or two years, frying tomatoes will make them more yang.

Our bodies always strive towards balance. If we eat strong yin food we afterwards crave for strong yang food. Meat is very yang, alcohol and fruit from warm southern countries are very yin. Salt is yang, sugar is yin.

Macrobiotics try to avoid eating strong yin or yang food. Thus they reach a balanced emotional state.

I always have some basic food in the house such as brown rice, miso soup, umeboshi plums, kuzu, whole oats, soy sauce and sea wheat. That's enough to balance extremes such as a bad tummy, sickness or constipation.

But it is not enough to start eating macrobiotic. You really have to listen to your own individual body in order to choose the right food.

Spoiling Time

Start with one to six weeks of spoiling yourself. Eat all your favourite foods, eat as much as you like too. Remember what you used to like as a child. Remember your favourite recipes and the places you like most for eating out. If you start feeling guilty, take the flower essence Pine. Rock water helps with strictness and perfectionism, Impatiens makes you slow down to enjoy the food properly.

Take lots of time to go shopping. Go to your favourite shops. Always buy the freshest food. Use your instincts and always buy things in abundance. Your inner child needs to feel safe and know for sure that there is enough food.

Take enough time to have tea in a corner cafe and read the paper. Once you have come home cook your food slowly. Sit down comfortably on a decent chair in a warm room to cut your vegetables. Put some music on as well. For eating choose your favourite plate or bowl and fork. Take plenty of time to eat and chew. It is good to eat without distraction such as TV, reading, talking. Do not pick up the phone while you are eating! Practise self-respect. Try to taste the food on your tongue and eat, chew and swallow it slowly, take a break and breathe. Find out if you really like the taste of the food. Only eat as much as you really want. Never think of finishing the plate just for the sake of it.

This first phase of the 'Loving yourself diet' is not just for people who want to loose weight but also for the ones who always eat what they are supposed to eat and what they think is good for them. It is for those who are always concerned about doing things right or wrong. They sometimes seem to miss their individual inner instinct or intuition to find the right choice. Cerato is the Bach Flower essence for that particular state of mind that many of us are familiar with.

The 'Loving Yourself Diet'

Loving yourself means being nice, patient, trusting and encouraging towards yourself. Quite often our inner relationship with ourselves is strict, full of hate and mistrust.

We usually automatically acquire the relationship with ourselves that our parents used to have with us as children. If we need to loose weight we might have overeaten because our parents did not give us enough real love. Food is a good substitute for love for couples and for children and their parents. If we haven't been breastfed and thus did not get our basic food from the very beginning of our life we might well sense that there is always something missing in our life but we might have forgotten what it was.

In order to fill this emptiness we might have started to always eat more than we needed. When children eat big portions of porridge at the age of two, the parents get used to this and think that the amount they eat would always increase. But there is actually a time around three or four, when they start eating much less and grow less. If parents are not aware of that fact, they might try to force the child to go on eating big quantities. Thus they might push their child into the habit of overeating.

There are many other conditions that can lead to overeating, and body orientated therapy might help a person to find out the true reasons for their overweight.

Making Choices

If you think that you have eaten as much and whatever food you like for as long as you like (about 1-8 weeks are recommended) you can gradually go over to part two of the 'Loving yourself diet'. You might be 'fed up' with a lot of things such as sweets, meat, cream and biscuits and that is good. As you gave yourself lots of time to eat and chew slowly, sit comfortably, without being distracted and use your favourite plate and cup some of your old habits might already have changed slightly.

Try to find yourself a counsellor or/and start writing a journal to review your daily life, especially talk or write about memories that come up, feelings and old habits. Express feelings such as anger, bitterness, fear and loneliness – preferably with the use of a cushion – in your therapy. Start having regular massage and go to a sauna every week. Any kind of movement such as yoga, keep fit, tai-chi, dance, walking, running, cycling and gymnastics are helpful with the process.

Artistic or musical expression can bring you more in touch with your feelings too. Start taking remedies such as Agrimony, Crab Apple, Alexandrite, Azurite-Malachite and Black Cohosh. Each of them can make you more sensitive about what you are eating.

The next stage in the programme would be to make choices. Try to find out about your own rules; What do you believe is healthy and good for slimming and what do you believe is not? Let's start with the drinks. We've got:

- black tea   – herbal tea
- real coffee – grain coffee
- fizzy drinks – mineral water

When you have breakfast you have the choice of white bread and brown bread, bread with chemicals or organic bread, sugared jam or sugar- free jam, milk and soy cheeses, cows', goats' and soy milk, butter and margarines with unsaturated fatty acids, white sugar or brown sugar, honey, fruit sugar, rice syrup or dried fruit.

You see now what I mean with making choices. Buy the two products and put them on the table. Allow yourself to try them both and then choose truly what you want to eat at a time. Try to make a choice from your belly, not so much from your head. I could imagine that after a while some of you might get a bit fed up with the unhealthy fattening options.Making real choices is something that not everybody is familiar with. Too often we have tried to push ourselves into doing something that our inner child has hated.

As lunchtime comes we might have a choice of either:
- tinned vegetables, frozen – fresh organic, biodynamic vegetables
- white rice and pasta – brown rice and pasta
- fat or red meat – lean meat, poultry or fish, soy meat or tofu burgers.

The more healthily you eat, the more you give your body what it needs and the less you want to eat.

A test has been made with three year old children. They were offered lots of different food. In the beginning they probably had more sweets than healthy foods, but after a while they all started to choose a very healthy and balanced diet.

It does work when you start to trust your very individual taste, as long as other basic needs are not missing. You only have to be patient. The time where you offer to yourself choices of food should last from one to four weeks. At the same time you are taking gem and flower essences and follow the above suggestions. Self-massage can be very helpful at that time. Stand in front of the mirror and try different clothes on. How do you want to look? Which clothes do you like and what would you want to look different? It is good to take time for those questions. After the stage of choices we will have a one-week diet.

I wonder how far you got with making food choices? I would like to offer you some help but not too much. If you are listening too much to me and not enough to yourself, things will always start going wrong. The most important step to becoming a 'conscious soul' is to start looking at yourself as a person who has all the wisdom of life deeply hidden inside themselves.

Let us start with breakfast. Let us assume that you usually have white toast with margarine and marmalade, a cup of coffee with white sugar and a bowl of cornflakes both with long-life milk (because it was convenient to buy those things from the corner shop) and an apple.

Let us imagine that you had two weeks of spoiling yourself and ate croissants with butter and expensive apricot jam, fresh coffee with cream and sugar, egg, bacon, baked beans, mushrooms and tomatoes and cream yoghurt with strawberries. If you were asked to describe a healthy breakfast you would say: Organic brown bread with healthy margarine and sugarfree jam, grain coffee (Barleycup, etc – there are many types) with soya milk and honey or fried tofu with baked beans on brown toast and a bowl of organic muesli with nuts, dates and fresh fruit, especially apples and pears.

The time of spoiling yourself might have had an effect on your eating already. You sometimes had indigestion afterwards or the taste in your mouth was uncomfortable after breakfast. For your choices you might have for your breakfast the following: Real coffee and grain coffee, milk and soya milk, white sugar and honey, white bread and organic brown bread, butter and margarine, fried bacon and fried tofu, sugared corn flakes and organic muesli with fresh fruit and nuts. You would take your time and try both options at the same time and decide which of them you would like more. What to you prefer? Real or grain coffee? White or brown bread? etc.

If people are able to keep a strict diet for a few weeks they will certainly lose some weight, but they will also gain it again later as soon as the discipline wears out. What we want to achieve are real living new habits of eating which the whole person likes and wants. They can only be acquired very slowly in everybody's individual way which is different for each person. These new habits will last much longer than any imposed diet.

Now I want to say a few things about dairy products, refined flour and white sugar. They all create mucus in the body. What is mucus? Mucus stops the energy from flowing. It can result from food, environmental pollution and chemical additives and from unexpressed emotions, just to name a few. It is also called 'waste products'. Mucus from cheese or white sugar can get stuck in the chest and create kind of a soft warm cushion as a substitute for love. Food often serves as a substitute for warmth, love and care. But all the sticky mucus we take in doesn't really belong to our body. It is a stranger and therefore it will always be in the way and inhibit the natural function of the body. Thus it has to be eliminated again.

As soon as the body has time and space it will start to get rid of the mucus. Everybody knows that mucus will be eliminated via our digestion or through nose, ears and mouth. If we collect too much mucus we might get a cold to help eliminate it. Mucus in the chest comes out as a slimy cough. Mucus, if not eliminated, tends to go deeper inside the body and stick around muscles to make them tense. The last place for the solidifying mucus is between the bone and a thin skin around the bone which is called periost.

Gerda Boyesen, the founder of Biodynamic Psychotherapy and Massage has invented the 'periost massage' where you mainly work on those blockages around the bones. Bones that are surrounded by this blocked crystallised energy will hurt when they are pressed and rubbed (as I have already mentioned in the chapters about hand and foot massage). Proper massage can eventually clean the bone and release the blocked energy. Slowly food specialists are accepting this knowledge but there are still many people who believe that they should drink a few glasses of milk every day to stay healthy and fit. But more and more people nowadays are starting to become sensitive and allergic to dairy products.

As a child I could not eat cheese. I hated the taste of milk and would never eat any chicken. In Bavaria people have lots of milk and dairy products. Mostly in the country people think that dairy products are very healthy. Dairy products contain lots of calcium, however, and it is not easy for people with calcium deficiency to get calcium from other sources. The healthiest dairy product, which I still have occasionally, is yoghurt with acidophilus bacteria. It has a beneficial effect on the digestion

Spend as much time as you like with making your choices. You will see that your food habits will very slowly start to change. But it can only happen if you really start to love and truly respect yourself more than you did before. That also means doing things in your own time in a balance position where you breathe and relax.

Once your stomach and belly shrink they need exercise and massage. When I was pregnant I oiled my belly everyday with olive oil and exercised my stomach muscles every day – especially after the pregnancy. That helped me not to get any stretch marks and keep my belly thin and firm all through the years. Massage your belly and stomach as deeply as possible. With the finger tips you can dig into the belly and work on the tonus of the intestines.

Try to soften the muscles if they feel too hard and try to strengthen them, if they are too soft and floppy. Pain can come from tension or inflammation. Pain from tension can be improved with deep massage, pain from inflammation should not be influenced with massage. It rather needs healing and holding to get better. Whenever you have time, breathe in and tense your belly muscles. Hold your breath and the tension for a while. Then breathe out and let go. Do this five to ten times a day. Once your belly feels empty and sensitive again you might not want to change this delightful feeling for all the food in the world. It is such a difference to being numb and insensitive.

Fasting is the best way to help you to get there. But fasting should be prepared by a one week-diet. The flower essence Crab Apple is especially suitable for preparing a fast. But the intake can cause in very few cases some side effects such as spots, excema and ulcers which are all ways the body eliminates waste products via the skin. Crab Apple can make you very taste sensitive. You probably will eat more selectively. Crab Apple can also make you feel cleaner inside your body. Thus you might get less affected by your environment. People who are very fussy about smells and dirt can benefit very much from taking this essence. It can help to create in us a very healthy attitude towards being clean inside and outside ourselves and as a consequence of that to feel more confident and less critical.

Diet Before the Fast

Before you begin with your weekend fast, you can follow a one-week diet. For example, one day's intake could be:

Breakfast: *Two slices of rice- or rye-bread with margarine, sugar-free jam or umeboshi paste or cooked whole oats with stewed apples or pears, roasted nuts, figs or dates and soy or rice-milk, bancha tea or barleycup with soy milk*

Lunch: *Cooked whole rice, millet or barley with two cooked vegetables with miso sauce or salad with a dressing made from olive oil, cider vinegar, soy sauce and fresh herbs*

Snack: *Oatcakes or ricecakes with tahini or sugar-free jam, bancha tea or barleycup with soy milk or fresh fruit*

Dinner: *Miso soup with fresh vegetables and seaweed, rye-bread or rice-bread with tahini or humus, stewed fruit with soymilk or soy dessert*

If you wish, you can also have a one-week fruit diet before you start with the fast.

Fast

The fast begins preferably on a Saturday morning. It is good to do the fast with a friend in the countryside. Put all the food away and avoid going to places where you have to watch people eat. Also avoid crowds, driving, traffic, television, smoke and noisy places. The fasting will make you more sensitive. You will like massages, sauna, bath, country walks and swimming.

During the cleansing the body will eliminate old waste products. As a result you might get headaches. Memories from the past and feelings such as anger, loneliness, grief and bitterness can easily come up too. Make sure that you will have someone to listen to you. Express yourself through writing, drawing, singing, dance and play. Have as much water, miso or vegetable broth and fruit juice as you like.

After two or three days break your fast slowly. Eat very little fruit or brown bread and chew it really well.

Diet After the Fast

Then again go on a one-week diet similar to the one before the fast. Enjoy your sensitivity and try to make it last for a while. Only eat the food you really like and do not overeat. Keep taking the crab apple for another two weeks. I am only making suggestions. Every person is different and has to find out for him/herself what they like.

Heal Your Mouth and Jaw

After having dealt a lot with eating, fasting and the 'Loving yourself Diet' we want to look at other issues connected with our mouth. In the introduction I have already mentioned that there is a close link between head and pelvis, between mouth and genitals.
There are exercises where you might be able to feel this connection directly. We will come to them later. The theory of the 'ring-muscles', especially described by therapist Paula Garbuck in her book *The Secret of the Ring-Muscles* is not just mentioning this close connection of mouth/throat and genital muscles.
She is referring to all the ring- muscles of our body as a system that works closely together.
Our mouth muscle is a so-called ring- muscle. There are ring-muscles around the throat, the intestines, the arteries and the genitals, just to name a few of them. All the ring- muscles in the body are working together like an orchestra. If we improve the tone of the mouth muscle, it will have an effect on the tone of the throat muscle and the other ring muscles.
If you exercise for example the mouth muscle in a special way, then after a while other ring- muscles start to move as well. Remember that it is essential for a muscle to be in a 'good tone' – that means not too tight and not over-relaxed. We can see people with lots of different mouth shapes. Some lips are very small and tight, others are full of fluid and too loose, others look a bit worn out like an old rubber band.
The shape of the mouth is slightly changing all the time. A mouth with a good tone has got the shape of a heart. Quite often people

with a heart shaped mouth stick out from the crowd and as you look at them you find yourself wondering if they have been singing, acting or practising any mouth exercises.

A lot of people – mostly women – smile too much. Of course in some professions it might be necessary to smile. Nevertheless, it is true that too much automatic smiling can wear out the mouth muscle.

Some people have a habitual smile and as soon as it goes, the corners of their mouth are hanging down and make them look depressed.

We often talk without using our lips enough to form the sound. Therefore it is a good exercise to start with pronouncing a poem by forming every syllable with shaped lips, as if a deaf person would have to be able to read the words from the lips. If your muscle tone is too loose, then this simple exercise might already give you the sensation of a togetherness of the lips, a sensation of security and safety. The tight 'O' where you tighten every bit of the muscle and hold the tension for a minute is the best sound for a loose tone.

Lip muscles that are too tight and thin need a big opening of the mouth instead. The best is to go from the big open 'lion's mouth' in very slow motion to the very tight 'O', and back again. After a few minutes of practising, stay in the 'in between state' and tighten and loosen little bits of the mouth muscle again and again.

Then practise an 'U' where you curl your upper lip around your nose (it is enough to work towards it) and support it with the lower lip. Hold this shape tight for a minute and then relax. Blow your lips with a 'brrrr' if possible. That is a good and relaxing exercise for trumpet players.

People who smile too much usually do not use words where they have to shape their mouth to an 'o', such as "go away","no, I don't", "I won't". They would rather say "yes" and "very nice" instead. Sometimes they smile while talking about something sad as well.

A smile is opening you up to your environment. You take the energy in and that means you are vulnerable. If you get hurt and you are still smiling it might be a good idea to use some words that close you down and push the world away from you, such as those mentioned in the last paragraph.

Some people have a body posture that invites others to drain or hurt them. It is good to be consciously open to the world and to take it in, when it is gentle, loving and safe. But if you are feeling tired, worn out or hurt it is time for you to close yourself down effectively. Quite often very old habits caused by parental or teachers' influences can be changed once you start noticing them properly. For example you might have been asked to smile at teachers as you were greeting them – but you don't really have to do that anymore as an adult. You can choose to smile when you want to. Of course, there are some people who never smile.

A good flower remedy for the ones who smile too much is Agrimony. And the ones who never smile might need cheering up with Mustard, Gentian, Wild Rose or Holly to express their hidden anger.

The following exercise, if practised in a relaxed way, might be useful for people who suffer from incontinence, indigestion, and for women who have given birth and suffer from too loose vaginal muscles. This exercise can help you to experience the close connection between mouth- and genital muscles.

Lie down on your bed. Have your legs up, heals touching the buttocks. Then start pronouncing the 'u' and the 'eeh' alternatively. Shape your lips like a comb as if you would say 'cheese' for the camera for the 'eeh' part of the sound. Tense the lip muscles properly. Do the exercise twice a day for five to ten minutes until you get the result you want.

Vocal Expression

I sometimes run voice workshops where we work with sound, breathing and massage for a whole day. I will only suggest a few exercises here. After having practised a few of the vowel sounds you might want to do a creative exercise now. If you are inhibited, you might find this one too difficult and would rather stick to some more precise instructions. In my voice workshops I always have to watch the people carefully and then decide if I am going to offer this creative exercise to them because it only needs one person to be inhibited in order to stop the whole group.

However, if you have been practising the 'moving your arms freely to music' exercise, you might like this one as well.

Babies are usually babbling all the time before they learn to say words. Young children still have this ability to use 'gibberish' or sing and hum along without words, as they are playing.

If you think that you are not creative, if you think that you cannot sing, dance or draw, if you think that you always have to be told how to do things, then this exercise is for you. But you might not be able to do it straight away. It might take you a few days or weeks to learn and you might need a safe space where you are alone and nobody can hear you. Do not think that this exercise is childish and do not underestimate it.

Lie down on a comfortable mattress and close your eyes. Then start to pronounce the vowels 'a', 'e', 'i', 'o' and 'u'. Imagine that you are a toddler and start to make sounds. Take your time and do not forget to breathe. Here are some guidelines for people who feel a bit inhibited:

Try to make a few of your favourite animal sounds. Then imagine that you are eating and make sounds – don't forget to use your tongue for this. Finish off by imagining that you are singing in a choir. Try to make your own individual sounds. Try to have fun. And afterwards you might want to be quiet for a while.

This exercise can release a lot of suppressed emotions. Therefore it is advisable not to go too far on your own. If you need help, contact me or another therapist who works with emotional expression.

Chanting the Vowels

This exercise can help you to centre yourself. Sit down on a cushion with your back straight and breathe. Visualise the spine and the chakras or energy centres. For the base chakra use the sound 'u' three times. Take a deep breath and chant the vowel as long as you can. It doesn't matter what it sounds like. Then go up to the hara, the chakra which is situated five fingers under your navel. Use the sound 'o' three times. Then move to the heart chakra with the sound 'a'. Move further to the throat chakra with the sound 'eeh' and shape your mouth like a comb. The last sound is 'e' for the third eye chakra, which is situated between the eyes. Then visualize the top chakra on the top of your head and be silent for a few minutes. Feel the energy moving upwards along the spine.

This exercise is like a meditation. It can clear the energy in a room within a very short time. Notice that there is no sound being used for the abdomen chakra. Notice that the sound 'eh' is different from 'e'.

Free creative expression is a natural skill that everybody has got. Of course some people can do those exercises straight away without any problems. For others it will take years to be able to relearn them. I personally believe that free creative expression can be the key for many people to grow into a new, different person.

That's why in my therapy I try to help clients, if they are interested, to get in touch with those exercises and to learn to be able to express themselves freely in different basic ways. Often being in a group can help to overcome inhibitions.

There are several basic types of creative expression. The first one is vocal expression of sound and words. The second one is expression with hands and arms. Creative movement as part of a dance, free painting and drawing, free writing of poetry or inspired writing, modelling with clay, wood or other materials are just a few of the different possibilities for creative expressions with arms and hands. The third basic way is creative expression with legs and feet. Of course free dance is the most important one.

In London there are dance events where you can dance freely – mostly without shoes. Those places usually prefer guests who do not smoke or drink alcohol. Children are usually welcome and do not have to pay. The music people dance to reaches from folk, jazz and classical music to 60's rock'n'roll and trance music. The five rhythms of Gabriele Roth have helped a lot of people to get in touch with their bodies and dance in a creative way – these might be worth investigating. There are some dance teachers who give individual lessons as well.

Once you are able to express yourself creatively in different ways you will feel much more free in other areas of your life as well.

At school we have always been told exactly how to do things right. Our natural ability to dance draw or sing without being told how to do it has thus been suppressed over many years.

Of course every one of us has been told very well what is right or wrong. We know too well how to critizise and how to be critizised. Thus the muscles in our arms, hands, legs, feet, mouth and jaw have become tense and stiff from too much inner and outer judgment. The only way to undo and relax them is probably to be able to create for yourself a space free of criticism.

Thus you can use one of the options for creative expression, which are named above to start making yourself a space free of criticism. At first you've got to be able to watch your mind very carefully to be able to catch yourself whenever you are judging yourself. The small judgments are usually easily overseen.

You don't have to give praise to yourself either because that could just be another way of judgment.

Get a big piece of paper and some nice pencils. Do not use crap material for this exercise but try to use your favourite pens and paper. Put some music on that means something to you. Make sure that you have got at least half an hour to spare without other people interrupting you. Sit down comfortably, preferably on the floor.

Start drawing without any concepts. Do not try to draw any particular things from your surroundings or from your fantasie. Try to free yourself from concepts. Try not to name your painted lines and do not find any interpretations. Just leave them free of any judgmental thoughts and call them your creative expression of that very moment and nothing else. Do not show them to anybody. It is good to draw a few pictures very quickly and think of something else in the meantime.

This exercise can be more difficult for people who have learnt or studied art and they probably think that they might not need to do it. But it is always worth trying for them because they might be the worst judges of all.

Helpful essences are:

- Larch for self-confidence
- Beech for being less judgemental
- Agrimony for self-expression
- Rock Water for accepting yourself more the way you are
- Impatiens for taking your time

Self-Massage of the Face

One of the best remedies to go to sleep is the massage of your own face, particularly of the forehead. But be careful because the massage of jaw and mouth can have the opposite effect and wake you up or even make you angry. In Biodynamic Massage we always think in terms of relaxing or provoking parts of the body. Either we are clearing things or we are stirring them up. If a client is already in an emotional state of tears or anger, I tend to give them a clearing and relaxing treatment. If they are in a good and balanced state, they often want me to help them to work on old and suppressed material and one way do do that is to give them a provocative massage.

Start your face massage in a lying position. Cover yourself to keep warm. Now massage your forehead from the middle above the nose with both hands towards the temples. The best is to use the fingertips of the three middle fingers. Use strokes and circular movements. At first explore the texture of your skin. Is it oily, dry or moist? Can you feel fluid cushions under your fingertips or does it feel bony? Fluid cushions want soft touch whereas bony structure might need a harder approach. Breathe through your open mouth while you are massaging. Do you remember what I wrote when I was describing foot and hand massage? What signs from the body are we looking for as a feedback for a good massage?

Deep breaths, sounds from the stomach, called peristalsis, electrical currents mostly in arms and legs, a meditative emptiness in the head, burping and yawning are just a few of the signs to watch out for. Massage your eyebrows with firm strokes and try to feel any small stony particles or fluid cushions under your fingertips. Imagine that you are cleaning and clearing the forehead and the eyes. You are helping the excessive waste products and the fluids to find their way out of the body via the digestive system. Massage the area under your eyes with soft movements from the nose towards the temples. This is an area where fluid cushions easily tend to develop.

So far this massage will help you perfectly to go to sleep. Practise it as often as you can to learn to know your face really well and to be able to massage other people's faces in the future.

People usually come with all kinds of vocal imbalances. Some women have a very high and childish voice. They usually do not breathe deeply enough so their voice cannot reach the deeper registers. It is possible through breathing exercises to deepen your voice. But a lot of people are not even aware of their imbalance. Men quite often prefer a female who is slightly childish, helpless and dependent in their behaviour. That makes them feel strong and needed (for protection). Some voices are too quiet and easily overheard. These people sometimes get attention because they speak so quietly. Of course this might not be true for a man. A man is usually supposed to have a loud voice. Some men speak far too loud and have to learn to tune in more.

Another problem arises if people speak too fast. Quite often bad speaking habits stem from early childhood traumas. One child always had to shout loudly to be heard, another one never had enough time to speak.

Everywhere we find a strong resistance to growth. Some foreigners seem to keep their accents because they sound funny or charming.

Even being able to have an image of ourselves as we appear to other people and knowing the impression they get of us is something we are often afraid to find out.

But once an imbalance is accepted and changed, a whole new world can open for this person. They might develop more self-confidence and find new friends, a different job and a new creative talent – who knows?

Quite often the throat seems to be blocked. People describe it as a feeling, as if they had swallowed an object. They sometimes have a constant cough, they seem to breathe very shallow or unevenly. Of course birth traumas quite often can be the deeper reason for this imbalance. Connective breathing and rebirthing can sometimes help to remember old traumas and it can help to practise breathing more deeply and rhythmically.

The jawbone tends to be stiff and blocked in lots of people. Some bioenergetics practitioners press the jaw quite firmly to enable people to scream, but I don't usually use this provocative method. Gerda Boyesen was the first one to teach me that it is much better to work with the feelings that are there or to give them patience time and space to come up. She made me believe that anything that is suppressed in the psyche, however long ago, will reappear when there is an accepting and receiving space for it.

I have spent lots of time at the dentist and the hygienist to strengthen my gums and prevent my teeth from falling out. I do believe that the inner child in us will, although numbed with injections, take notice of all the unpleasant and frightening events that take place in our mouths. I often compare them to roadworks. There is a lot of anger constantly stored in and around the jaw. Lots of things we could not say or express are bottled up in that region. Thus by going through dentist and hygienist treatments we are revitalising old feelings of anger and frustration and they sometimes come up a few hours or even up to a week after the treatment.

Gems, Gem and Flower Essences for mouth, jaw and neck
- Snapdragon, Celadine, Dill Aquamarine helps to soothe sore throats
- Lapis Lazulii helps to correct speech imbalances
- Chrysocolla, Turquoise, Sodalithe help with throat blockages
- Agrimony is a bach flower for vocal expression and relaxation
- Heather helps to speak less
- Cosmos helps with speech coordination.

Self-Massage of Mouth, Jaw and Neck

This kind of massage can be provocative. That means that it might bring up anger and prevent you from going to sleep within the next few hours. So please only use it when you are in a safe, grounded space and preferably have a friend or therapist nearby to help.

Find a comfortable place to lie down and cover yourself with a blanket. Then with the fingertips massage your jawbone from the inner side of the eye towards the ear. Follow the shape of the bone, as if you would polish it. Try to feel the consistency of the bone and the muscles and tissue attached to it. Painful areas need more attention. Watch out for the `telephone answers' from within the body such as a deep breath, stomach sounds, electrical currents, yawning and burping.

Then massage the area under your nose carefully. Feel the gums. Give some extra attention to the 'smiley' corners of the mouth. Try to massage the place where the upper and lower jaw is connected with extra pressure. Massage the stubborn chin. It usually feels insensitive and blocked. Try to massage the jawbones from underneath along the neck.

Very carefully massage the front of your neck where the adams apple is situated. This is a very sensitive place, but by exploring it very carefully maybe for the first time in your life you can overcome some of your basic fears. Try to relax the throat with gentle massage.

If you are more experienced you can try to make yourself slightly cough and make the mucus come out from your eyes and nose. This

kind of gentle elimination can help you not to get a cold.
Massage your lips with the thumb and index finger. If they are full of fluid you might get fluidic sounds. After this massage you might be fit for the vocal expression exercises that I have described in the previous chapters.

Now massage the vertebrae upwards to the beginning of the hair line with your fingertips in a circular movement as if you were polishing them starting with the vertebra at the base of the neck. It will probably take a while for the body to respond to your massage with the usual feedback (sounds from the intestines, deeper breath, electricity like movements, burping and the tendency to yawn and stretch, images and memories). Usually five to ten minutes of numbness are to expect then the area will open up.

Be patient and use enough pressure. Then 'pluck' the string of muscles and tendons on the right and left side of the neck like a guitar string hard enough to feel it clearly relaxing. Then massage the neck with the whole hand.

Keeping Your Sacrum More Sacred

Now we arrive at the final destination on our journey through the body which brings us to the sacrum and the lower back, an area which causes plenty of distress to many people.

Sacrum, Pelvis and Lower Back

After having found a brilliant picture of the sacrum I started to think to which bones in our head the sacrum and the pelvis were related. German Philosopher Rudolf Steiner's most important message is probably that we have lived on this earth before and that we are going to come back again.

Especially since I came to England I have had a huge number of past life memories in the form of dreams, glimpses and images.

Those experiences made it clear to me, that I have been living here before and that I have been meeting many people under different circumstances too.

Rudolf Steiner says that our trunk of this life will form the head of our next life. What an exciting idea!

So which bones of the head are going to be related to the sacrum and the pelvis?

I thought first that it was the epiglottis, the roof of the mouth. But I was a little wrong. L.F.C. Mees' book, *Secrets of the Skeleton* helped me to find out.

The answer is:

The temporal bone (pelvis) and the sphenoid bone(sacrum)

The sacrum is a triangular shaped bone lying between the 5th lumbar vertebrae and the coccyx. It consists of 5 vertebrae that are fused together to form wide lateral wings. It articulates on each side with the bones of the pelvis thus forming the sacroiliac joint.

'Sacrum' in Greek 'heron osteon' bone = sacred bone. It has the name from its sacrificial use. The word originates from 75-200 BC.

Up to now I have not been able to find out, how this bone has been used for sacrifices and I would be pleased if one of the readers could tell me more about it.

While practising connective breathing I have experienced some visions, which I'd like to share with you.

The ones that have read my story *Tobias and the Augenblick* might remember that Tobias during a dream found himself in the valley of the hidden feelings. There he met the cuddlesome cats that wanted to be stroked.

All the animals he met were symbolic for areas of the body where feelings had been blocked. The cats were symbolic for the belly and pelvis area.

In my visions I saw the ovaries as two cats, a male and a female one standing like 'sphinx 'on both sides of the gate. The 'sacrum' I saw as the gate to the sacred ground.

In Michael Ende's book *The Neverending Story* a little boy had to pass two sphinxes whose eyes nearly killed him before he could enter the gate and finally come to the castle of the princess.

The so-called 'Gundalini energy' is rooted within the base chakra not far from the sacrum.

That's from where the 'dragon' can rise and the energy can move upwards along the spine and awaken the chakras, the energy centres of the body.

There are similarities between the genitals and the mouth, as I have mentioned before. With the mouth 'we give birth' to the word.

The word is like a being that we go on creating as we speak. (Look at the first chapter of St.John's gospel about the word.)

The holy grail and the 'lance' can be another symbol for the sexual act being transformed through metamorphosis into the mouth and the tongue (or the word.)

The Numbness of the Pelvis

I have found out that for a lot of my clients the lower back area around the sacrum is either painful or numb. Usually pain as a warning signal helps us to do something about it. But what about numbness?

Hardly anybody can feel the sweet sensations around the sacrum any more. We have lost them because we are too much in our head thinking. Many of us have big bellies and we do not move anymore as much as we used to when we had neither cars, aeroplanes and washing machines, nor radio or television. And we mostly breathe far to shallow.

Feeling numb can be frustrating! It creates a sensation of emptiness. Thus we are looking for stronger stimuli and sensations. Some want to see horrible movies, drive fast cars, or eat concentrated food such as white sugar and flour or filet steaks.

We are no more happily waving our arms around, running across the meadow to get thrilled. We need more than that to get excited.

We have lost the paradise of our childhood. And how can we get it back again?

How can we sensitise our numbed body again?

I have already mentioned in the introduction that, while studying psychology in Munich I had singing lessons and bioenergetic sessions. I had a very high and thin voice and I always wanted to sing deeper and with a bigger volume. My singing teacher asked me to breathe into my lower back and hold the breath for a while. He also taught me panting, a breathing technique which is used for pregnant mothers to help them with the birth process, I received my first deep lower back massage and became aware of my numbed lower back and the tension I was holding there for the first time in my life.

The tension was mainly situated around the sacrum. Deep massage and breathing exercises helped me to free the tension and thus deepen my voice. If you imagine the body as being like a double bass you would think that vitalising the lower half of the back would enlarge the 'sound body' and deepen the breath and the voice. It would also increase people's sexual sensitivity. They would be more able to feel the orgasmic energy stream going up the spine.

Muscles are living beings. Like a rubber band they can get too tight or over-relaxed. Tense muscles can cause pain, over-relaxed muscles can make you feel numb.

Massage can help to restore the natural tone of a muscle. But can we always touch those muscles? What can we do if they are deep inside the body?

I have already mentioned the 'ring-muscle exercises' by Paula Garbuck. They are also called 'Sphincter Gymnastics'

I have always imagined that there was a connection between the mouth and the genitals. About 15 years ago, when my friend showed me a leaflet with the title The secret of the ring-muscles I was very interested to find out more about it.

I rang the practitioner and he offered to teach me a set of exercises. I had to lie down on a mattress with my knees bent and was asked to open and close my eyes in my own rhythm for about 10 minutes. Then my mouth started to move and I made involuntary grimaces. I expected that the teacher would ask me to stop but he was welcoming all the involuntary movements of my body. Eventually my legs started to move. I kicked my pelvis on the floor and I began to tighten and relax my bladder muscle. After about 30 minutes of involuntary moving I stopped. I felt very relaxed and satisfied. It was as if my whole system had been renewed and energized.

I had 10 sessions with my teacher and then he had to go back to Israel. He was a bit disappointed because he didn't experience much response to his leaflet. The title was probably a bit too scary for the English.

He said that Paula Garbuck had written a book on the subject but he didn't think it had been translated into English yet.

I asked every Jewish person I met if they could help me to get hold of this book – without any success.

Only 3 years ago a woman came to my house for therapy. She had experienced 'Sphincter Gymnastics' with Paula Garbuck and she gave me a translated copy of her book. She also gave me the phone number of a teacher who was living in London.

For a whole year I worked with Ayelet and benefited enormously. I might go back to see her again. She is a very fine classical singer and gave me singing lessons too.

'Sphincter Gymnastics' is based on the fact, that we have voluntary and involuntary sphincters. We can activate the involuntary ones with using the voluntary ones through special exercises.

In the so-called 'Rem-phase' during sleep we move our eyes rapidly. These eye-movements, a kind of blinking are one of the basic exercises in Paula's system (as mentioned before.)

There is a parallel between those exercises, the primitive reflexes of a baby and the involuntary activities of our body.

There is a law that all the sphincters or ring-muscles work simuiltaneously and affect each other.

A smoker's oral ring-muscle is usually over-relaxed. The smoker uses the cigarette pressed between his lips partly to create a tightening effect of his mouth muscle. That helps him to concentrate better and give him satisfaction.

The lower sphincters (anus and bladder) of a smoker usually are over-relaxed too. If they are not working properly they can cause in the smoker a feeling of dissatisfaction and emptiness.

The functioning of the two lower sphincters has a deep effect on the whole body. Contracting and relaxing them in a regular rhythm can help many other sphincters to improve the 'muscle-tone'.

Paula Garbuck's method has helped to improve or heal lower back pain, arthritis, impotence, haemorrhoids, prolapse of the uterus, lumbago and many other symptoms. It is worth reading Paula's book or having therapy sessions with a certified instructor.

My sister in Germany is a gymnastic teacher. She knows everything about the relationship between the head (mouth) and the pelvis (genitals). She teaches pregnant mothers what they call 'Beckenboden Uebungen' (pelvis exercises).

Alexander teachers are helping people to become more sensitive about the energy movement up the spine with exercises and creative visualisation.

I have mentioned before that pregnant mothers and people with big bellies can experience a constant forwards and downwards pull on the spine. Thus the muscles along the spine will have to carry a lot of weight. They will tense up and eventually a layer of tissue will form around the tense muscles. The muscles will constantly hold the tension. As a response to that people stop breathing deeply into the lower back. The area can become painful or insensitive and numb. The breath might become more shallow and the voice might get higher and thinner. This process can also take place with hereditary deformation of the spine and of course whenever we develop a bad posture

All this can take years to develop. There is a strong tendency in the body to keep it alive and in balance. But through constant strain it will eventually give in and develop a safety armour that will keep it functioning. The person has to pay for it by becoming less sensitive. A few years ago I wrote a song where I compared this process with the fakir sitting on his board of nails. Two children pass by and the boy says: "I wouldn't mind being like him, then I would not feel it if father hits me." The girl answers: "But you wouldn't feel mum's kisses and cuddles either." The song ends with the verse:

"And our false smile shines miles ahead,
we are racing nummed on vast streets through the city,
between movies, star fighters, Hot Dogs and TV
and if someone has still kept their senses alive and is still amongst us
they should pack their things and leave as soon as possible,
because it seems that we are all dying on the board of nails
and nobody is aware of it."

Sleeping Beauty in Grimm's fairy tale sleeps in a tower for 100 years. Then the prince has to come through the thorny rose hedge with his sword and awake her with a kiss. Quite often, people who find their life force again through massage, healing, flower essences and other means will feel exactly like Sleeping Beauty waking up from a deep, long sleep.

About Breathing

Feeling the lower back in a vibrant and joyful way is a luxury. Most of us adults have to work 'hard' to get the feeling back which we experienced as a child in this area. Our breathing has usually become very shallow. We breathe into the upper chest if we are lucky but we hardly breathe any further down into lower chest, belly and lower back. The following exercise can help you to deepen your breathing. Lie down on your bed on a hard mattress. Put your hands on your upper chest and try to breathe into the upper chest in such a way that you can feel the chest lifting under your palms. Breathe three times with an open mouth and then move your hands onto your rib-cage. Breathe three more times into the rib-cage and feel it widening like an accordion. Then move the palms to the top of your belly. Breathe into the belly three times. Move the hands now onto your lower back. Some people might find it difficult to breathe into that area. Their lower back might be feeling numb. Move your hands a little bit up on both sides of the spine to where the kidneys are. Breathe three times into the kidneys. Imagine that you are a butterfly spreading its wings. Try to move further up to the shoulder-blades. You might have to turn your hands round to reach the upper back.

The next place to breathe into is the neck. Then move to both sides of the skull and then to the cheeks. Finish this exercise by breathing into the upper chest. Now lie on your right side and feel the spine with your left hand all the way from the neck to the coccyx. You probably have to miss out a few vertebrae.

In his book *Healing Sounds*, Jonathan Goldman describes the break between in-breath and out-breath as a still-point where the human body is locked in resonance with itself. Scientist Itzhak Bentov believes that the body creates a wave form that operates at about 7.8 cycles per second. This is believed to be the resonance frequency of the earth and at this still-point while we are locked in resonance with ourselves we are also locked in resonance with the earth.

The life energy contained in breath is supposed to be sacred. The

Hindus call it 'Prana' and in the Orient it is called 'Chi' or 'Ki'. In Hebrew it is called 'Ruach' which means 'Spirit'. Reich called it 'Orgon'. For massage and therapy it is the best thing to allow the natural breath to deepen just by breathing through the mouth, watching it and allowing the breathing muscles to relax.

In yoga, breathing through the nose is usually recommended. It helps to keep emotions down and find a calm and clear space. I have already described how important it is to learn how to breathe into the lower back. I have called this way of breathing 'butterfly breathing'.

'Connective Breathing' is easy to learn but should not be used without a helper or a therapist. Eventually they can bring you into a state of ecstasy but before that you might have to go through all kinds of painful feelings and memories from childhood or even past lives. Breathing and emotions are closely related to each other.

I believe that every suppressed breath in any part of the body can be remembered and re-lived just by using connective breathing. As we breathe in actively and rhythmically into our upper chest and let the out-breath go naturally we eventually get in touch with all the experiences in the past, where we have suppressed our breath and our emotions.

Sometimes fast breathing is recommended. Many people will go to sleep straight away in the beginning of practise sessions. Slowly they can learn to stay awake and alert a bit longer.

All the mucous in chest and lungs which has been collected through the suppression of feelings, through environmental pollution and the consumption of the wrong food has to come out again via digestion or through coughing, spitting, crying and other methods of elimination.

This way of hyperventilation can cause numbness and a light paralysis of mouth and hands. This does not last long. After a while the body relaxes again and goes back to normal. But I try to avoid this from happening because people tend to get frightened. This is one reason why beginners should have a trained helper at their side.

They can wake them up as well and assist them with the expression of feelings. They can give them hugs, cushions, water to drink, tissues and a 'spitting bowl' if needed and listen to them kindly. The breathing sessions can start with five minutes and then last up to 1 hour. Afterwards people are usually exhausted and need a rest and a quiet and safe space. Group sessions are not always a good solution because there are never enough 'mummies' to hug and console the people who get into distress. Used in a modest way the connective breath can deepen the awareness, relax and help to go to sleep.

Some of you will not feel anything at all or go to sleep most of the time. Then you should leave it and try something else – for example have deep rolfing sessions or practise bioenergetics.

Being in balance also means to breathe in a balanced way. I am a jazz-pianist and I love playing New Orleans Jazz. I experience 'Swinging' as a phenomenon where the rhythm is not as accurate as an electronic beat. 'Swinging' for me is a natural rhythm where the heart and the consciousness are alert.

The point of stillness between inbreath and outbreath where we are one with the earth energy needs to be consciously experienced by each musician. Then the musicians are present with all their energy. They are not distracted by thoughts or feelings of fear, false pride, boredom or anger. They are not impatient but they seem to have all the time of the world. They are in touch with their own inner time that has nothing to do with clocks and watches. Children are like that and and so are people from early cultures. In the west most of us have to learn it again from scratch. That is the only way to become a truly creative person.

Breathing and sex go closely together. Energy can be exchanged in a circular movement. To get to this experience you need to be 'in touch' with your partner, breathe in a little bit later then your partner and breathe out just a split of a second later than your partner. Thus you can enter the circular breathing which can move through the whole body in a wave of ecstasy. This experience can also occur when we are feeling one with nature, with the moon, the sun, the sea or with a tree.

In his book *Orgasm* Jack Lee Rosenberg writes that the way we move can influence the way we breathe and the way we feel vice versa. With different bioenergetic exercises for both individuals and partners he helps people to increase their energy level and work on sexual problems.

Felix Riemkasten, in his book *The Alexander Technique*, recommends one not to draw the shoulders up and to breathe out as completely as possible. We usually do not take enough time to breathe out properly. But we should not push ourselves in any way during this expanded outbreath. And once it is out he recommends we should have a little rest in between and wait until the new breath really wants to come in again. Only then we give way to the new breath and thats all. In our time many people suffer from impatience and nervousness. Thus they never breathe out properly and they always breathe in far too early.

John Diamond describes the lung meridian as the meridian of humility. A balanced meridian implies tolerance, humbleness and modesty in an indivual. Intolerance, disdain, contempt, false pride and prejudices occur when the meridian is unbalanced. The lung meridian is our prime meridian. It is involved in early child development.

Thorwald Detlevsen in his book *Illness as a Way* sees breathing as tension and relaxation – in german 'Spannung' and 'Ent-spannung'. Breathing is giving and taking. In Latin 'spirare' means breathing. We feel 'inspired' by something as if we have received an idea together with our breath.

In breathing we have to exchange the air with other people. We are thus forced to share. Some people develop asthma because they are too sensitive to share the air with others.

If we cannot breathe freely any more, we feel trapped and imprisoned. Too much freedom and responsibility can create fear of breathing in and out. The breathing muscles contract with fear.

As soon as they begin to keep the tension our breathing becomes inhibited. Our breathing becomes more shallow and the body does not any longer receive enough breath to be vital amd alive. Thus it slowly starts to disintegrate and go numb or ill.

In her book *To the Light,* Polish clairvoyant Lilla Bek describes various breathing exercises to use for balancing the different chakras.

Lilla is a friend of mine and she has taught me many things during her courses in Tekel's Park, a nature's trust park in Camberley, Surrey. She can see auras and tune in with whales and other animals.

Self-Massage of the Back

Lie down in a comfortable position on your right side. Try to feel a 'bunch of muscle strings' on the left side of your spine. Carefully roll your knuckles across the strings in both directions, What can you feel? This bunch of muscles is sometimes not easy to locate. A layer of tissue, the so-called armour might surround it. This body armour, as Wilhelm Reich the German psychotherapist has named it, serves as a de-sentisitizer. We went through a lot of emotional pain in our life and the body in order to survive had to develop this armour. If we manage to create a safer environment for ourselves we can start slowly to let this armour go and become a more sensitive person.

Try to massage this bunch of muscles with the fingertips or the knuckles of your left hand from the neck all the way down to the coccyx. Try to feel the very beginning of pain and relax into it by breathing with an open mouth. These muscles might have been in a tense spasm for years and it might take a bit of pressure to ease the tension.

Then roll onto your other side and apply the same kind of massage with your right hand on the right side of your spine. Being massaged on your back by another person is without any doubt a much easier and more relaxing thing but you can't always get it when you need it. Self-massage is the best way to learn about massage because you will get a feedback from inside. Some people lie on hard stones or other firm objects and feel the pressure on their back as a satisfying sensation. Others use one of those electric massagers which sometimes can be better than nothing.

Another useful way of feeling the lower back is exercise. Lie down on the floor and bring your knees towards the chest. Hug your knees with both arms. Roll to the right and left side. This can be like a spine massage. If you have difficulties bringing your knees further towards your shoulders do not force it. It should not hurt. Those with fairly flexible spines can now bring their legs across the head and if necessary support the lower back with both hands, but be ever so careful and don't force anything. The legs do not have to be straight. They can be bent and lie on both sides of the head. The legs could also rest on a chair or lean against the wall. The main thing is to stay in this slightly uncomfortable position for a while. The stomach is squeezed and therefore the breath will go into your lower back. This breath is called alpha breath. Babies breathe like that and experience a lot of bliss. The alpha breath relaxes and can bring you into a pre-dream stage where you might see visions.

Once you have had enough move very slowly back by visualizing your spine as a snake and taking one breath per vertebra (as a rule of thumb). This exercise can be more fun if you put some nice music on. Bring your feet back to the ground next buttocks. Lift your spine and lower back up and then push the coccyx down to the floor a few times. Make a sound with an open mouth. This exercise is helpful for expressing anger and impatience. But be careful and do not overdo it. Now bring the coccyx up and move your back up very slowly thinking of one vertebra for one breath. Once the whole spine is up try to stay there for a while. The very flexible ones can even stand on the top of their head and touch the heels with both hands. This is the opposite to the first exercise. The spine is bent to the other side. Go back very slowly. Then have a rest.

Bioenergetic exercises have been developed by Wilhelm Reich, Alexander Lowen and J.Rosenberg. They are all body-orientated psychotherapists and they have written a few very good books on bioenergetics. You can improve your breathing, work on emotional expression and get some better grounding by practising them regularly.

There are groups at the Open Centre in Old Street, London (East West Centre). Once you have learnt how to breathe into your lower back and feel it as a support area you have to work on keeping in touch with it all by moving, bending and sitting the right way. Always keep your spine straight. If you want to pick something up from the floor move with your buttocks slowly down to a squatting position and then pick the object up. Put your clothes on by sitting on the floor or on a chair. Take your time and breathe. You are nobody's servant and therefore you do not have to rush anything. Choose a chair with a 90-degree angle on the back. Keep your spine straight while you are sitting. Do not cross the legs as this will stop the energy flow. It is a good habit to change your sitting position every so often. Experiment with sitting on one leg or have one bent leg with the foot on your chair. These positions have the advantage that they will support your spine but can't be held for long. Kneeling on a chair or sitting like a Buddha is another option. Working on the floor might be the best solution if possible. If you have to sit on a soft sofa, make sure that you support your lower back beyond the kidneys with a hard folded cushion or with your fist, I usually use my coat or jacket on the dentist's chair. Make sure that working surfaces are not too high or too low. Put one leg on a chair to support the spine if necessary. That is good advice if you wash your clothes in the bath. Make sure that you sleep on a hard mattress. If you slowly alter your bad habits your lower back will soon improve its condition.

Our body wants attention especially in the areas that are out of balance. If we give this attention to the body as we would give it to a small child the body will be happy and work for us without 'moaning and groaning'.

Flower and Gem Remedies for the lower back are:
- Oak for strength and grounding for people who work too hard
- Elm for grounding you in difficult times in your life
- Holly to help you express anger and overcome it
- Centaury for the weak willed dependent kind of people to strengthen their will Vine for the ones who are too dominant and hardened in their attitudes
- Rock Water for being soft and gentle with yourself (eases rigid muscles)
- Dandelion to relax muscle tension (can also be mixed with massage oil.)

Gem Stones for the lower back are:
- Tiger's Eye
- Copper
- Amber
- Jet
- Black Tourmaline
- Fire Agate
- Obsidian
- Pyrite
- Fluorite
- Amazonite
- Boji Stone.

Both the stones and their essences can help with back pain, grounding, expressing and overcoming anger and feelings of heaviness and irritability.

Sexual Issues

Sexual issues are closely related with the area around pelvis and sacrum as a 'cradle' for the genitals.

Quite often I get clients with sexual problems.

Reichian Therapy, Sphincter Exercises, Biodynamic Massage and Flower and Gem Essences can often help people to enjoy sex more.

In the sixties a lot of noise was made about achieving orgasms as if they were the main reasons for having sex. Nowadays people are more careful and take into account that 'the way to reach a goal' should be at least as important as the goal itself. People are more encouraged to enjoy the foreplay. Usually we find mostly men rushing through the foreplay either full of impatience and 'sexdrive' to have an orgasm or wanting to get it 'all over and done with' as soon as possible.

A lot of British people are very shy about sex. Mixed saunas are still rare and you find the few women who go there wearing bathing costumes. Massage has still got a bad reputation in many people's views and that bad reputation keeps them away from it.

The island position of Great Britain could be one explanation why the English seem to need so much space around them and find it more difficult to get close on a bodily, mental and emotional level than the people on the continent. Children being sent to boarding schools away from home from five years onwards only makes things worse.

The lover and the friend or housewife and mother often have to be two different people. They often cannot be one and the same person. Maybe the idea of sex having to be something 'bad' or at least 'secret' or 'forbidden' is one reason for this phenomenon.

Sexual problems with couples

One difficulty that often arises is the lack of interest in sex in one partner. The more people can feel their bodies in a pleasurable way the more they can usually enjoy sex. Self-love is the basis for a healthy sex life. Other important factors are usually too much hard work (especially computer and office work tends to keep the energy stuck in people's brains), not enough joyful movement and play, too much television and overeating just to name a few.

Early potty training, sexual abuse and traumas, physical ailments can all contribute to lack of sexual interest in a relationship. Biodynamic massage for both partners can often renew the sensitivity in the body by releasing blocked sexual energy especially in legs, knees and around sacrum and pelvis. Practising deep breathing can loosen blocked energy and free repressed feelings and memories. Counselling is then very helpful for expressing feelings and talking about taboos. Gem and Flower essences when mixed and prescribed individually can help to a big deal to improve sexual communication between partners whereas sphincter exercises can help some people with impotence and frigidity.

In the sixties, Masters and Johnson, American therapists, were developing a useful programme to help people with sexual problems. A lot of questionaires had to be filled out and then the couple was usually encouraged to slowly start touching each other in non-sexual areas. This process lasted a few weeks to raise the sexual desire in the partner who had difficulties in getting turned on. Clients who were suffering from early abuse would be shown slides of naked bodies of the other sex or they were asked to imagine scenes they were afraid of in a vivid way. Then at the same time they tried with breathing and muscle exercises to fully relax their body. Sometimes couples were encouraged to try new positions where the woman could stroke herself at the same time.

Therapy for couples has always been easier than therapy for singles because they can always work together on their problem. But if a client cannot reach an orgasm at all, it is usually easier for them to learn to reach it by ways of masturbation. From there they can start to practise with a partner if possible.

Masturbation is important for both men and women and it can enable them to reach their full sexual potential. Just the fact that there is no English word for this activity, which sounds just as pleasant as it is shows already that masturbation is fully connected with feelings of guilt, of being bad and unacceptable. Thus it is usually performed in an unloving and quick way. There are very few people who can caress themselves slowly in a loving and gentle way. They are usually women.

For women there seem to be three different kinds of orgasms –

the clitoral orgasm can be reached by touching the clitoris in a rhytmical way. It is the orgasm for 'virgins'. Once the woman has had intercourse with a man she usually develops more the 'vaginal' orgasm. For some women this orgasm is often experienced as deeper and more fulfilling than the clitoral orgasm.

Twenty years ago people were writing articles where the vaginal orgasm was denied as a 'myth'. The last few hundred years have been full of sexual repression – mostly for women. Thus a lot of women never experienced any orgasms or only clitoral orgasms. The anal orgasm is not only satisfying for gays. People who overcome their prejudices can enrich their sex life. 'Anal' personalities (people who have problems to give things away) usually have tension in their intestines and anus muscle. In Norway doctors have found out that massaging the anus muscle and thus relaxing the muscle tension can be very helpful with haemorrhoids and other similar ailments. Women who want to develop the vaginal orgasm can practise this with a candle. The tonus of the vaginal muscle can be relaxed – either tightened or widened- in this way. It is good to breathe with an open mouth and then to try to hold the candle with the vaginal muscle. The vaginal or P-muscle can be trained on the toilet by holding the urine for a few seconds before urinating. Once we get a feeling for the P-muscle we can practise to hold and relax it a few times a day. If the P-muscle is too loose, intercourse can be unsatisfying.

The 'T' spot is situated about five centimetres on the upper side of the vagina (inside). Stimulation of this spot can help women to reach an orgasm. Also voluntary tightening and pressing of the vagina muscle combined with vocal expression or deep breathing can loosen the muscle tension and reach to further fulfilment.

'Ring muscle exercises' developed by Paula Garbuck are described in the chapter about vocal expression. For more information read Paula's book. Mouth muscle and vaginal and anal muscle are connected and the muscle tone of the sexual muscles can be improved with mouth exercises.

In the chapter about breathing I have described exercises from the book *Orgasm* by Jack Rosenberg. This book can be very helpful for people with healing their sexual problems. It mostly contains bioenergetic and breathing exercises.

'Connective Breathing' can be another basic tool for relaxation and overcoming sexual inhibition.

I have already mentioned how important it is to stimulate and sense the lower back muscles around kidneys, coccyx and sacrum. If they are sensitive we can feel the orgasmic energy going all the way up the back in a wave of ecstasy. The same is true for loosening the tension in the upper legs, knees and calves to be more able to feel the sexual energy streaming down the legs.

Earlier on I have described how you can enter the circular breath and feel one with a partner or with nature. Once you can breathe in a circle you might prefer this orgasmic experience to sexual orgasms (this might be a way the angels can feel orgasmic without having intercourse.)

As sexual problems usually are a very delicate subject it is difficult to write about them in general ways. It will be much easier to deal with them in individual therapy sessions.

But sexual therapy still seems to be in its childhood. There is still no reliable way to help everybody to experience a full orgasm. All the taboos about sex, especially in this country, are making things more difficult.

Gems and their Essences for Sexual Difficulties:
- Disturbed Sexuality: Garnet, Ruby, Rhodonite and red Jasper (to massage the belly below the navel)
- Impotence: Ruby, Red Jasper, Garnet or Rhodonite (to be put on the base chakra regularly in the evening for 20 minutes)

Sexual Disorders:
- Atacamite strengthens the genitals and eases gonorrhoea
- Copper strengthens the sexual organs
- Diamond can act as a mild aphrodisiac, it can also help to ease sexual dysfunctions with a psychological cause
- Dark Opal was used in Lemuria to open the sex chakra. It can ease sexual depression and help people to become truly sensitive
- Garnet (Spessartine) is used as an elixir to help with sexual diseases and psychological problems
- Gold, Copper and Silver essence can be taken together to balance sexuality
- Fire Agate can connect the sexual and heart chakra to work closer together
- Chrysoprase can open the sexual chakra and increase fertility in both men and women
- Fluorite can help with sexual frustration
- Gold Garnet (Spessartine), Loadstone, Magnetite, Dark Opal, Platinum, Silver, Spinel, Rubellite and Tourmaline can help to release sexual problems from childhood
- Lapis Lazuli, Dark Opal, Clear Quartz and Ruby essence mixed can help to transform sexual energies into creative expression

Flower Essences:
Impotency and Infertility
- Avocado can sometimes help with frigidity and impotency. It stimulates the sensitivity in the hands and makes people more able to enjoy touch.
- Bells of Ireland can revitalize vaginal fluids and increase fertility
- Blackberry and Fig can enable people to get out of their mind and more in touch with their body
- Mallow, Mugwort and Squash improves fertility and increases sensitivity.

Sexual Diseases:
- Papaya
- Squash

Aphrodisiacs:
- Avocado
- Mullein
- Papaya
- Petunia
- Pomegranate
- Spice Bush
- Watermelon
- Banana helps men to identify with their feminine nature and negate macho behaviour

Australian Remedies:
- Body Odour: Dog Rose, Five Corners. Billy Goat Plum
- Candida: Spinifex. Kangarooh Paw
- Cystitis: Dagger Hakea, Bottle Brush
- Cysts: Stuart Desert Rose, Mountain Devil
- Fallopian Tubes: She Oak, Spinifex
- Frigidity: Billy Goat Plum, Wisteria, Red Helmet, Flannel Flower
- Herpes: Stuart Desert Rose, Billy Goat Plum, Spinifex
- Impotence: Crowea, Flannel Flower, Five Corners

Californian Flower Essences:
- Self-Confidence and acceptance of the body: Manzanita, Larch
- Possessiveness in sexual relationships: Bleeding Heart, Pink Yarrow, Centaury
- Repression of sexual desire: Rock Water, Californian Pitcher Plant, Easter Lily, Hibiscus, Manzanita, Sagebrush
- Negative or destructive relationships: Black Cohosh, Holly
- Overcoming fear of intimacy: Sticky Monkeyflower, Poison Oak

- Sexual shame: Basil, Crab apple, Pink Monkeyflower, Purple Monkeyflower, Pretty Face
- Hardening of sexual forces after trauma, shock or abuse: Dogwood, Evening Primrose, Mariposa Lily
- Depletion of sexual forces: Lady's Slipper, Olive
- Sexual aggression and verbal hostility: Tiger Lily, Snap Dragon, Black Cohosh, Centuary Agave, Scarlet Monkeyflower
- Integration of sexuality and spirituality: Alpine Lily, Basil
- Sexual addiction: Basil, Chestnut Bud, Fairy Lantern, Morning Glory
- Confusion about sexual orientation: Calla Lily

It is not easy to write about sexuality because it is so comprehensive, People usually feel very vulnerable about sexual issues and in individual therapy it usually takes a few sessions before they start talking about sexual problems. Thus I can only touch the 'tip of the iceberg' of many problems. Any further work would have to be accomplished in individual therapy sessions.

Energy in Balance

Here we will focus on the two sides of the brain. The two hemispheres of the brain connect via a kind of beam called 'corpus collossum'. The left side of the brain is linked with the right side of the body and vice versa. Hands, eyes and ears are connected with the contra lateral half of the brain too. With the right side of the brain we hear music, listen to poetry, touch and smell.

We receive information in a holistic way in patterns and symbols. With the left side of the brain we think, speak and listen in an analytical, rational way. We analyse, write and create logical structures. Here lies our sense of time.

Thorwald Dethlefsen in his book *Illness as a Path* explains that according to the task we are accomplishing one side of our brain always dominates us. Via the beam or bridge of the brain there is always an exchange of information going on. Of course we would not be 'whole' if we only had one side of the brain. Nevertheless it seems as if the left side of the brain runs most of our present world. Rational, analytical and concrete thinking seems to be predominant and time always plays a big role in people's lives.

Dethlefsen writes that most of the things we usually critisize as irrational, occult and fantastic are simply part of the ability to look at the world from the other side of our brain. This often-suppressed shadow side of us can become important whenever we are in danger. Then our human nature often changes to the use of the right side of the brain. Once analytical thinking cannot help any more we can benefit from the ability of the right side to get a holistic overview and put us into a space where time does not seem to exist any more. The two poles seem to compensate each other and therefore we cannot use the two sides of the brain together at the same time. As humans we are forced to use one side of the brain after the other and thus create rhythm, time and space. Healing and initiation can both be a pathway leading from polarity to unity. We can only overcome the polarity that seems to keep us in a space where we identify with the egoistic human nature when we do not separate ourselves from the universe. First the ego needs to grow and then it has to die otherwise we cannot become part of everything. To overcome the polarity we need to change the domination of one side of the brain into using them both at the same time. The beam or bridge needs to become more and more permeable and two brains need to grow into one. The subjective conscious has to unite with the objective unconscious. The universal wisdom of this step from polarity to unity can be found in Taoism as yin and yang. The hermetics talk about the marriage of fire and water or the unification of sun and moon. The two snakes of the 'caduceus' are symbolizing the two polar energy streams called ida (female) and pingala (male) that try to overcome the canal in the middle called hashumna. The polarity of our consciousness always forces us to decide between two possibilities but we can only achieve one at a time. In order to find the right decision we have to judge and critizise. The only step that helps us out of this dilemma is the insight that there is no good or bad no right or evil. Every judgment is therefore subjective. These things have to be deeply understood if we want to find a balance in life on different levels.

Flower and Gem Essences
Australian Flower Essences:
- Bush Fuchsia for dyslexia, clarity in speaking, stuttering
- Sundew, Isporgon for brain imbalances.

Californian Flower Essences:
- Amaranthus stimulates thymus and pituitary glands, helps with clear thinking and disruptive dream states
- Comfrey increases physical coordination
- Mugwort heals damage to the right brain, nervous tics or twitches can be eased.

Gems and Gem Essences
- Picture Agate
- Amber
- Copper
- Coral
- Diamond
- Gold
- Rutilated Quartz
- Silver.

Massage of the Head

After having learnt in other chapters how to massage the face and the neck I will describe to you how you can massage your skull.
Sit or lie down in a comfortable position and breathe through your mouth into the upper chest.
Gerda Boyesen used to talk about 'hills and valleys' on the skull. Hills are swollen areas containing fluid and often sensitive to touch, valleys are mostly dry and depleted areas that need to be vitalized. 'Valleys' usually need strong pressure whereas 'hills' can respond to very light touch. I still tend to add pressure on swollen sensitive areas by pressing them and lying on the back to use the weight of the head as pressure until the 'bubble' bursts sometimes with a loud watery explosive sound similar to the blockages behind the ears.
Very light touch can stimulate sensitive brain waves and cause lots of different sensations, images and responses on other places of the body. For this kind of work you need time and patience. Massage on the back of the head and the forehead is usually the best way to go to sleep. It is good to start with neck massage to relax the neck muscles and vertebrae first. Aurawork on the head is very calming too.
'Spirals' can be drawn out of the top of the head to reconnect with the spirit. 'Padding' of the aura and balancing by holding your hands on the aura above the ears can have a relaxing effect. Spirals can be moved out from the ears as well (see the chapter about the ears).
In `Brain Gym' we find a selection of exercises, which are taught in

primary schools in Germany to help the children overcome learning difficulties. There are exercises for 'middle line movement' helping the pupils to be more able to cross the middle line between the right and left side of the brain, stretching exercises and energizing exercises. Inability to cross the middle line can lead to Dyslexia and learning difficulties.

Finally I only want to mention a few exercises .These exercises are also good for a stiff neck.

'The Lazy 8s'
An exercise where we draw a big figure eight with our left arm in the air or on a black board at least three times.

'Double Doodle'
We draw lines on a black board with both hands simultaneously. Head and eyes should be allowed to move. Some of the exercises are commonly used in gymnastic classes:

'Neck Rolls'
We breathe through an open mouth and gently roll the neck from one side to the other in a circle. This exercise helps with earthing, centering and relaxes the central nervous system.

'The Energizer'
In yoga they call it 'Cobra': We lie on the front, the hands and forearms under the shoulders. Then we breathe in and slowly lift head, neck, chest and arms. The throat has to stay open, the energy should move upwards.

'Breathing into the Belly'
The hands are both crossed on top of the belly. A rhythm of three counts in, three counts holding and three counts breathing out is recommended. The palms should be lifted by the breath.

References

Life Energy, John Diamond Dodd, Mead & Co, New York 1985
Healing Sounds, Jonathan Goldman, Element 1992
Total Orgasm, Jack Lee Rosenberg, Random House Inc 1973
Eigenbehandlung durch Akupressur, Gerhard Leibold, Falken Vedag 1977
To the Light, Lilla Bek with Philippa Pullar, Unwin Paperbacks 1985
Krankheit als Weg, Thorwald Dethlefsen, Rudiger Dahlke, C. Bertelsmann Verlag 1987
Self Healing, The Secret of the Ring Muscles, Paula Garbourg, Peleg Publishers 1994
Bioenergetics, Alexander Lowen, Penguin Books 1976
Secrets of the Skeleton, L.F.C. Mees, Anthroposophic Press, 1980
Bewegung ist Heilung, Simon Pressel
Die Alexander Methode, Felix Riemenkasten, Karl F. Haug Verlag, Heidelberg 1967
Gem Elixiers and Vibrational Healing Vol 1. 1985, Gurudas-Cassandra Press, San Rafael, Ca.
Flower Essence Repertory, Patricia Kamiresley and Richard Katz, Earth Spirit Inc, 1994
Flower Essences and Vibrational Healing 1983, Gurudas-Cassandra Press, San Rafael, Ca.
Elementarwesen, Marco Poogacnik, Knaur 1995
How to gain knowledge to the higher worlds, Rudolf Steiner,
Australian Bush Flower Essences, Ian White, Findhorn Press 1991

Individual Sessions and Workshops with Gabriele Gad
Biodynamic Massage,
Counselling and Flower Essences
020-7735-4513 London SW8
Website: www.gabrielegad.co.uk

Individual Sessions for Sphincter Gymnastics and Singing lessons
Ayelet Amitai
mobile 079 613 47069, tel. 8444 9031

If you would like to know more about:
- Biodynamic Body Psychotherapy
- Biodynamic Massage
- Biodynamic Therapists
- Experiential Introductory Weekends
- Short Course in Biodynamic Massage
- Professional Training for the Diploma in Biodynamic Psychotherapy

please contact

THE LONDON SCHOOL OF BIODYNAMIC PSYCHOTHERAPY
Tel/Fax: 0700 079 4725
Email: enquiries@lsbp.org.uk
Website: www.lsbp.org.uk

Made in the USA
Columbia, SC
02 December 2024